Social Drivers of Health

Implications for Clinical Practice

Editors
Sandra F. Braganza, MD, MPH, FAAP
Kevin P. Fiori, MD, MPH, MS, FAAP

With a Foreword by Andrew D. Racine, MD, PhD, FAAP

American Academy of Pediatrics
DEDICATED TO THE HEALTH OF ALL CHILDREN®

American Academy of Pediatrics Publishing Staff

Mary Lou White, *Chief Product and Services Officer/SVP, Membership, Marketing, and Publishing*
Mark Grimes, *Vice President, Publishing*
Carrie Peters, *Editor, Professional/Clinical Publishing*
Grace Klooster, *Editorial Assistant*
Theresa Wiener, *Production Manager, Clinical and Professional Publications*
Amanda Helmholz, *Medical Copy Editor*
Peg Mulcahy, *Manager, Art Direction and Production*
Soraya Alem, *Digital Production Specialist*
Sara Hoerdeman, *Marketing and Acquisitions Manager, Consumer Products*

Published by the American Academy of Pediatrics
345 Park Blvd
Itasca, IL 60143
Telephone: 630/626-6000
Facsimile: 847/434-8000
www.aap.org

The American Academy of Pediatrics is an organization of 67,000 primary care pediatricians, pediatric medical subspecialists, and pediatric surgical specialists dedicated to the health, safety, and well-being of all infants, children, adolescents, and young adults.

While every effort has been made to ensure the accuracy of this publication, the American Academy of Pediatrics does not guarantee that it is accurate, complete, or without error.

The recommendations in this publication do not indicate an exclusive course of treatment or serve as a standard of medical care. Variations, taking into account individual circumstances, may be appropriate.

Statements and opinions expressed are those of the authors and not necessarily those of the American Academy of Pediatrics.

Any websites, brand names, products, or manufacturers are mentioned for informational and identification purposes only and do not imply an endorsement by the American Academy of Pediatrics (AAP). The AAP is not responsible for the content of external resources. Information was current at the time of publication.

The publishers have made every effort to trace the copyright holders for borrowed materials. If they have inadvertently overlooked any, they will be pleased to make the necessary arrangements at the first opportunity.

This publication has been developed by the American Academy of Pediatrics. The contributors are expert authorities in the field of pediatrics. No commercial involvement of any kind has been solicited or accepted in the development of the content of this publication. Dr Iman Hassan has disclosed a financial relationship with Baxter Pharmaceuticals as a consultant. Any other disclosures were reviewed and determined not relevant to the work related to *Social Drivers of Health: Implications for Clinical Practice*. Disclosures are reviewed and mitigated through a Conflict of Interest process that consists of reviewing pertinent information which is then used to decide what action is required to maintain content integrity. There may be instances where no action is necessary. This process has been approved by the AAP Board of Directors.

Every effort is made to keep *Social Drivers of Health: Implications for Clinical Practice* consistent with the most recent advice and information available from the American Academy of Pediatrics.

Please visit www.aap.org/errata for an up-to-date list of any applicable errata for this publication.

Special discounts are available for bulk purchases of this publication. Email Special Sales at nationalaccounts@aap.org for more information.

Printed in the United States of America

9-517/0125 1 2 3 4 5 6 7 8 9 10
MA1177
ISBN: 978-1-61002-791-5
eBook: 978-1-61002-792-2

Cover and publication design by Peg Mulcahy

Library of Congress Control Number: 2024944053

AAP Reviewers

Council on Community Pediatrics

Council on Environmental Health and Climate Change

Contributors

Editors

Sandra F. Braganza, MD, MPH, FAAP
Director, Social Pediatrics Program
Department of Pediatrics, Children's Hospital at Montefiore
Department of Family and Social Medicine
Associate Professor of Family and Social Medicine and Pediatrics
Albert Einstein College of Medicine
Bronx, NY

Kevin P. Fiori, MD, MPH, MS, FAAP
Vice Chair, Community Health & Engagement
Division of Community & Population Health
Department of Pediatrics, Children's Hospital at Montefiore
Associate Professor of Family and Social Medicine and Pediatrics
Albert Einstein College of Medicine
Bronx, NY

Contributors

Rachel Stein Berman, MD, MPH, FAAP
Assistant Professor of Pediatrics
Division of Academic General Pediatrics
Albert Einstein College of Medicine
Children's Hospital at Montefiore
Bronx, NY

Zoe Bouchelle, MD, MSHP, FAAP
Instructor of Pediatrics
University of Colorado School of Medicine
Denver, CO

Earle C. Chambers, PhD, MPH
Professor of Family and Social Medicine
Director, Division of Research
Albert Einstein College of Medicine
Bronx, NY

Michaela Domaratzky, MD
Clinical Assistant Professor
NYU Department of Pediatrics
New York, NY

Carol Duh-Leong, MD, MPP, FAAP
Assistant Professor of Pediatrics
Division of General Pediatrics
NYU Grossman School of Medicine
New York, NY

Arvin Garg, MD, MPH, FAAP
Professor of Pediatrics With Tenure
Founding Director, Child Health Equity Center
UMass Chan Medical School
UMass Children's Medical Center
Worcester, MA

Iman Hassan, MD, MS
Associate Professor of Medicine
Division of General Internal Medicine
Albert Einstein College of Medicine
Bronx, NY

Alejandro Hermida, MD, MSc
Pediatric Emergency Medicine
Children's Hospital Los Angeles
Los Angeles, CA

Isuree N. Katugampala, MD, MPH
Attending Pediatrician, General Pediatrics
Maimonides Children's Hospital
Brooklyn, NY

Yonit Lax, MD, FAAP
Chief, Pediatric Community Health
Maimonides Children's Hospital
Assistant Professor, Clinical Pediatrics
SUNY Downstate Health Sciences University
Brooklyn, NY

Jana C. Leary, MD, MS
Faculty of Medicine
Harvard Medical School
Boston Children's Hospital
Boston, MA

Samantha Levano, MPH
Senior Research Coordinator, Community Health Systems Lab
Division of Community & Population Health
Montefiore Children's Hospital
Albert Einstein College of Medicine
Bronx, NY

Michael J. Luke, MD
Fellow, Pediatric Hospital Medicine
Children's Hospital of Philadelphia
Philadelphia, PA

Hemen Muleta, MD, FAAP
Instructor of Pediatrics
Department of Pediatrics
Albert Einstein College of Medicine
Bronx, NY

Milani Patel, MD, FAAP
General Pediatrician
Durham, NC

Dana Sanderson, MD
Assistant Professor of Family and Social Medicine and Pediatrics
Montefiore Children's Hospital
Bronx, NY

Jenna Scholnick, MD, FAAP
Assistant Professor of Family and Social Medicine and Pediatrics
Division of Academic General Pediatrics
Montefiore Children's Hospital
Bronx, NY

Marc F. Shi, MD, MSc
Assistant Professor of Medicine
Division of General Internal Medicine
Albert Einstein College of Medicine
Montefiore Medical Center
Bronx, NY

Radhika Teli, MD
Assistant Professor of Pediatrics
Department of Pediatrics
Albert Einstein College of Medicine
Montefiore Children's Hospital
Bronx, NY

Andrew Telzak, MD, MSc
Assistant Professor of Family and Social Medicine and Pediatrics
Albert Einstein College of Medicine
Bronx, NY

Aditi Vasan, MD, MSHP
Assistant Professor of Pediatrics
Division of General Pediatrics
Perelman School of Medicine
Pennsylvania & Children's Hospital of Philadelphia
Philadelphia, PA

Dedication

Through decades of insightful discussions about social drivers of health and social justice, we dedicate this book to all the residents and faculty of the Social Medicine Program, especially the Social Pediatrics Residency Training Program, the oldest residency program in the United States focused on caring for children in underserved settings.

We also dedicate this book to all our past and present patients whom we have the honor of caring for. Their trust and resilience and the stories they share have taught us more than any textbook could.

SFB and KPF

Equity, Diversity, and Inclusion Statement

The American Academy of Pediatrics is committed to principles of equity, diversity, and inclusion in its publishing program. Editorial boards, author selections, and author transitions (publication succession plans) are designed to include diverse voices that reflect society as a whole. Editor and author teams are encouraged to actively seek out diverse authors and reviewers at all stages of the editorial process. Publishing staff are committed to promoting equity, diversity, and inclusion in all aspects of publication writing, review, and production.

Contents

Foreword

The major portion of any "cure" is a social matter which has broader and more fundamental implications than the actual medical and surgical treatment of a case.
Ephraim Bluestone

There is just no point in treating rat bites—and ignoring the rats.
H. Jack Geiger

Pediatricians have known since the dawn of the discipline that social conditions strongly influence the developmental trajectory of children's health. What the World Health Organization has come to define as "...the conditions in which people are born, grow, work, live, and age, and the wider set of forces and systems shaping the conditions of daily life"[1] frames the foundation on which health status is constructed.

The term social *determinants* places rhetorical emphasis on a purportedly causal set of relationships. When we seek to account for variation in the incidence of disease among different populations, this framing has considerable merit. Social inequities visited on identifiable groups of people, whether differentiated by race and ethnicity, income level, geographic location, preferred language, or other characteristics, can reliably be traced forward to health status differentials. That is why these social conditions have come to be termed social *determinants.*

Yet we also know from empirical observation that estimates of the percentage of variation in health outcomes of individuals accounted for by these social factors is imprecise. Health outcomes at the individual level are notoriously unpredictable. Indeed, that is why individuals seek to purchase insurance—to mitigate against this uncertainty. Although their explanatory power for a given individual may be more modest than the term *determinant* would suggest, the influence that these features exert on the health of individual children and their families is nevertheless undeniable.

What is more, the work we accomplish in the examination room takes a back seat to these more primary influences. The explanatory power of the receipt of health care services in accounting for variation in health outcomes is quite limited, a realization that should occasion the adoption of a justifiable posture of humility on the part of physicians.

And yet, there is much that pediatricians can do in their practices to identify and address the needs arising from the lived social experiences of their patients and families. And that's where this volume comes in. The editors have crafted a comprehensive toolkit of valuable resources and practical advice drawing from their extensive experience in the field. Beginning with essential definitions that distinguish structural determinants, social risk factors, and health-related social needs, the authors go on to provide important context to emphasize the link between the work that can be done in clinical practice and the upstream conditions that this work is designed to address.

With illustrations of useful screening instruments, the organization of effective multidisciplinary workflows, specific considerations that pertain to the most prevalent social needs likely to be encountered in practice, and observations on future directions including training of the next generation of practitioners and planning for the inevitable disruptions that attend individual families as well as entire communities, this compendium covers a wide range of topics. Pediatricians may engage with the content as a whole or may pick and choose among the chapters to harvest those approaches most meaningful to their individual circumstances.

Approaching their task with a combination of rigor and humility, the editors have assembled, in their words, "...a series of evolving best practices for how to address [social drivers of health] in real-world clinical practice." The 2 most important words in that statement are *evolving* and *real-world*. The incorporation of social needs screening into pediatric practice is still in its infancy, so more work will need to be done to refine the approaches outlined in this volume. As this necessary work proceeds, however, pediatricians throughout the country will be able to avail themselves of this valuable resource, and the children and families they care for will be the better for it.

Andrew D. Racine, MD, PhD, FAAP
American Academy of Pediatrics President-Elect
System Senior Vice President and Chief Medical Officer
Montefiore Health System
Executive Director
Montefiore Medical Group

Reference

1. *Integrating the Social Determinants of Health Into Health Workforce Education and Training.* World Health Organization; 2023

Acknowledgments

We would like to thank the leadership of Montefiore Health System for their groundbreaking vision and dedication to Social Medicine and its transformative impact on the Bronx community and beyond. In particular, we are deeply indebted to Dr Peter Selwyn, chair of the Department of Family and Social Medicine, whose unwavering support and encouragement were instrumental in making this book a reality. Additionally, we would like to acknowledge and thank Dr Michael Cabana, chair of the Department of Pediatrics, for his steadfast commitment to our efforts.

SFB and KPF

I am thankful to my daughters, who inspire me to make the world a better place, and my husband, who has been an exemplary father, husband, and dedicated physician. Thank you to my parents for their unconditional love and guidance and for teaching me how hard work and sacrifice can make dreams come true. Last, thank you to my Social Medicine classmates, my mentors and colleagues who have been role models on how to address social justice and health equity.

SFB

I am deeply grateful to my family for their unwavering support throughout this journey. Their love, encouragement, and belief in me have been the foundation of all my professional aspirations. I would also like to express my sincere gratitude to my mentors and colleagues, both locally and abroad, whose guidance and expertise have been invaluable. Their dedication to this work has provided me with direction and inspiration.

KPF

Part 1. Foundations

CHAPTER 1

Introduction

Sandra F. Braganza, MD, MPH, FAAP, and Kevin P. Fiori, MD, MPH, MS, FAAP

Health is driven by more than just health care

Social drivers of health (SDOH), also referred to as *social determinants of health,* have been the focus of our collective professional careers, including educational, scholarly, and administrative pursuits both in the United States and around the world. As we conceived and planned this book, there were a series of key questions that were critical to consider before embarking on this process. Essentially, we needed to be clear about the *why, who,* and *how*—with emphasis on *who* was going to use the book. Knowing there are textbooks on the subject, we decided to create a resource to support the busy clinical teams that, for example, are treating patients with uncontrolled asthma whose family's bathroom is overrun with mold and mildew, trying to follow up with patients who cannot make appointments because of transportation barriers, or providing nutritional guidance to patients who are at risk for pediatric obesity but do not have access to nutritional foods.

Why do we need a book about the SDOH for clinicians?

Health is driven by more than just *health care.* In recent analyses, the United States continues to invest twice as much in health care expenditures relative to peer nations yet continues to lag in key population health metrics, such as infant mortality, life expectancy, and chronic disease prevalence. Simply put, we are not getting a return on our investment. As a result, we believe that the US health care system is experiencing a long-overdue paradigm shift. One might even refer to it as a *reckoning* that explicitly acknowledges the lack of investments in health disparities, social spending, and structural barriers to care that in turn drive poorer health outcomes for all.

The concept that a person's health is influenced by factors that exist outside the walls of our health systems, emergency departments, hospital beds, or clinics is neither new nor surprising to clinical teams that care for patients and their families. Health care professionals have been working for hundreds of years with the reality that a person's health is determined by more than just the provision of health services. Addressing the varied economic, social, and environmental conditions as well as addressing racism confronting the communities we serve is part of our framework for practice. Furthermore, there are numerous innovative and novel programs that have been developed to address these SDOH. But that is where the problem lies, as these programs are exceptional and extraordinary rather than commonplace and standard. Despite our understanding that social factors influence a person's health, clinical medicine has not traditionally focused on these SDOH as a deliberative and formal competency in the same way that fluency in comprehensive physical examinations is required.

Paradigm shifts are difficult in health care. What occurs during such a shift is an avalanche of new articles, pilot studies, policy statements, and programs—enough information and resources to overwhelm any part- or full-time practitioner. This can be not only a tremendous opportunity to improve care but also a confusing and time-consuming endeavor. At the time we are writing this book, there is an abundance of resources such as policy statements, guides, review articles, and research, but our belief is that there is not a clear *gold standard* for integrating social care into health service delivery but rather a series of evolving best practices for how to address SDOH in real-world clinical practice. We planned and curated this book, authored by experts in the field, to provide a compass for the busy practitioner, with the goal of providing a foundational tool to navigate this shift. Our authors all have real-world experience in developing best practices and advancing our field.

Who is the intended audience for this book?

Because social needs affect patients at the family level, this book is not just about caring for children and adolescents but also about caring for their parents, grandparents, or other caregivers (eg, aunts, uncles, other relatives). This book has relevance for those busy clinicians with an ever-increasing clinical burden who are now also trying to address another issue for the family, such as food insecurity or financial difficulties. We designed this text as a countermeasure to prevent discouragement, despair, and indifference and as a tool for inspiration, growth, and improvement. This text is neither an exhaustive list nor a step-by-step guide on how to address health-related social needs (HRSNs) in clinical care. We humbly acknowledge that the SDOH that affect our patients are neither straightforward nor resolvable within a 15-minute visit. The structural forces that often lead to what manifests as food insecurity, for example, are complex, and we are under no illusion that this text can solve those problems. Awareness and acknowledgment of the issue are not only required but insufficient for progress. So, this book was designed *not* (although, we hope, is still relevant) as a resource for the typical audience (eg, researchers, advocates, or policymakers who are entrenched in health equity issues) but rather for the Health Center team at a Federally Qualified Health Center, the busy private practice, or a rural community health center. We devoted several chapters in Part 1, Foundations, Chapters 2 through 4, to provide background for the busy clinician, or clinical team, who is committed to providing excellent clinical and social care for patients and their families.

How should one use this book?

As previously mentioned, we designed this book for the clinical setting; therefore, we anticipate that our busy clinician may not have time to read the book in chapter order. Hence, the chapters are designed to stand alone, and the reader may note some repetition of key concepts. The inclusion of key concepts and key points in each chapter allows the reader to rereview critical information or jump to pertinent sections within each chapter. Chapters are enhanced by the inclusion of figures and tables throughout as well as some resources to obtain additional information as needed. The book is divided into 3 parts. Part 1, Foundations, includes summaries of background and context (Chapter 2), existing guidelines and policies (Chapter 3), and screening approaches that can be used in the clinical care setting (Chapter 4). This part is an asset for anyone who is new to the concept of SDOH and HRSNs. Refer to Chapter 2, Social Determinants of Health: Historical Roots, Trajectory, and Nomenclature for the 21st Century, for an explanation of the distinction. It also serves as a useful review for those looking for a succinct summary of best practices.

Part 2, Social Drivers of Health, dives more deeply into a discrete number of social needs categories designed to provide background, best practices, and practical advice to the busy clinician. Please note that the focus is on the most prevalent social needs reported by patients in our collective institutions. These will include financial resources (Chapter 5), housing and the built environment (Chapter 6), and food insecurity (Chapter 7). It is not intended to be an encyclopedic review of each possible social need or a catalog of all possible social needs categories that patients report. In our experience, the system change(s) that address one social need category are often applicable universally, and we will review this on a practical level in Chapter 8, which focuses on interventions.

Part 3, Future Directions, is devoted to forward thinking around this topic, with chapters exploring training the next generation of clinicians (Chapter 9), disruptions and policy (Chapter 10), and future directions (Chapter 11). We wanted to provide the reader with ideas and concepts that will advance this field, although anticipating future directions is an imperfect science.

Because our experiences are subjective, there will undoubtedly be gaps in what could be covered in one text. But our goal is to produce a book that clinicians see as a way to improve patient care. We also invite our audience to review the many American Academy of Pediatrics (AAP) publications (eg, policy statements and books) addressing the SDOH and to join the many committees, councils, and sections of the AAP to partner in this discussion. We hope this text contributes to our current paradigm shift and brings health care closer to recognizing the SDOH as a standard pillar of clinical practice.

CHAPTER 2

Social Determinants of Health: Historical Roots, Trajectory, and Nomenclature for the 21st Century

Andrew Telzak, MD, MSc; Earle C. Chambers, PhD, MPH; and Samantha Levano, MPH

While awareness of the importance of social determinants of health (SDOH) has grown over the past 2 centuries, commensurate spending on social care programs has not. Building on the foundational works of Frederich Engels, Rudolf Virchow, W.E.B. Du Bois, and Salvadore Allende, the World Health Organization codified the SDOH framework in their Commission on Social Determinants of Health. Within this framework, important distinctions exist between the intermediary social causes of health and the distribution of these causes, which are driven by the larger structural determinants of health. A focus on the SDOH has recently gained traction within health systems through screening for health-related social needs (HRSNs). There is a strong evidence base supporting this work; however, large gaps remain in our understanding of the implementation challenges across complex health care delivery systems. While screening for and addressing HRSNs is a necessary step for health systems to address the intermediary social causes of health, upstream interventions requiring multi-sectoral policies and approaches are critical to reduce health inequities.

CHAPTER 2

Social Determinants of Health: Historical Roots, Trajectory, and Nomenclature for the 21st Century

Andrew Telzak, MD, MSc; Earle C. Chambers, PhD, MPH; and Samantha Levano, MPH

Introduction

The study of the nonmedical factors influencing health can be traced to the mid-19th century, in the work of Friedrich Engels and Rudolf Virchow in Europe, W.E.B Du Bois in the United States, and Salvador Allende in South America. The World Health Organization (WHO) continues this work with its Commission on Social Determinants of Health, which provides an important framework to understand the layers and interconnectedness of social causes of health. This chapter discusses the individual social causes of health outcomes (the intermediary determinants of health, such as living and working conditions and food availability) that are clearly delineated from the structural causes (such as the criminal legal system and the institution of racism) that determine health inequities. What follows is an examination of the suggested first step to integrating social care into medical care: screening for and addressing health-related social needs (HRSNs). But HRSN screening and navigation interventions alone are insufficient in the larger struggle to address health inequities. In fact, pairing these interventions with multisectoral approaches, as laid out in *The U.S. Playbook to Address Social Determinants of Health,*[1] is critical to tackle the structural causes producing inequitable health outcomes in our society.

Historical Context

The concept of health as socially determined is not new. In the mid-19th century,[2] Friedrich Engels unambiguously called attention to the living and working conditions among working class communities in England in 1845 as a root cause of illness and early mortality. During that same period, Rudolf Virchow, a German physician, identified poverty and lack of education as the main causes of a typhus outbreak in Upper Silesia in 1848. In the late 19th century, W.E.B Du Bois characterized racial health inequities, in particular how disparities in tuberculosis outcomes reflected the different social and environmental conditions in which Black people and white people lived.[3] In the 1930s, Salvador Allende, as the minister of health in Chile, identified poor sanitation and poor housing and working conditions as the main causes of illness for most Chilean people. Drawing on this historical context, the WHO emphasized the need to address the social causes of health in their landmark *Declaration of Alma-Ata* on primary health care in 1978.[4] In this statement, they defined *health* not only as the absence of disease but also as a complete state of physical, mental, and social well-being. The WHO has since codified the social causes of health as the *social determinants of health* (SDOH), "the conditions in which people are born, grow, work, live, and age, and the wider set of forces and systems shaping the conditions of daily life."[5]

In the half-century since, our understanding of the SDOH and the drivers of health inequities has continued to grow and evolve, with new emphasis placed on integrating social care into clinical practice.[6] Many regulatory agencies and academies now endorse the need to screen for and address the SDOH within routine medical care.[7] There is also growing evidence documenting deficiencies in population-level spending on social care in relation to health care. Compared to other high-income countries, the United States spends significantly less on social care and more on health care.[8,9] Within the United States, states that have a higher ratio of social care to medical care spending have also seen significantly better health outcomes than those spending less on social care.[10] In addition, social care spending in the United States has largely focused on individuals 65 years and older.[11] As such, worse health outcomes in states with lower investment in social care may be linked to the disproportionately lower investment in families with young children and individuals active in the workforce.[12,13] Investment in social care continues to be an evolving landscape, as do the science and nomenclature surrounding the SDOH. To begin to understand the current state of the science of SDOH and the role health systems can play in the integration of medical and social care, it is necessary to define the currently accepted language and frameworks for the layers of social causes of health.

World Health Organization Commission on Social Determinants of Health

The WHO Commission on Social Determinants of Health[14] provides a useful conceptual framework to understand the complex relationships between many of the terms frequently used to describe the social origins of health (**Figure 2-1**). Although the term *social determinants of health* is often used as a catchall phrase, we must understand and define the more specific nomenclature frequently used to describe the distinct relationships and causal mechanisms at play. Many of the SDOH that are often screened for and addressed in the clinical setting (eg, living and working conditions, food availability) are defined in this framework as *intermediary determinants of health*. Behavioral, biological, and psychosocial factors influencing health outcomes can also be thought of within this category of intermediary determinants of health. Taken together, these intermediary determinants are also referred to as the *social causes of health*.

Although everyone is affected by these factors (for better or worse), their distribution is inherently inequitable in our society. The reasons for this inequity are multiple and complex and require an understanding of the intersections between power, context, and identities that determine social stratification. Within this framework (**Figure 2-1**), we see that upstream factors that determine the distribution of social causes of health are defined as the *structural determinants of health inequities*. These include the socioeconomic, political, and cultural context and the socioeconomic position of individuals and families.

Social Causes of Health (Intermediary Determinants)

The intermediary determinants have been linked to health outcomes for close to 2 centuries and can be thought of as affecting everyone, shaping health outcomes for all individuals and communities. They are not inherently positive or negative and can be experienced as either social assets or social risks, depending on the circumstances. For example, 2 children may experience housing stability very differently, but both would be impacted by this as a social cause of their health. A child whose family owns its home may consider their housing stability a *social asset,* while another child whose family has moved within the shelter system in the past year may consider their housing instability a *social risk.* For both children, housing stability is inextricably linked to their overall health and well-being.

To understand how these social causes of health are affecting individual patients and their families in the health care environment, considerable effort has been put into the development and implementation of screening tools to measure HRSNs. Although the terms *social determinants of health, social risk factors,* and *health-related social needs* are at times used interchangeably, there is growing consensus around a clear distinction between these terms.[15,16] In contrast to the intermediary determinants of health (or *social causes of health,* as defined earlier in this chapter) that are neither positive nor negative and can be defined at a community level, *social risk factors* are defined specifically as adverse, measurable individual-level SDOH. For example, housing stability may be a risk or an asset as a social cause of health and can be defined at a community level through a variety of different metrics.[17] An individual child or family reporting that its housing is unstable, however, would be considered to have this as a social risk factor.

Health-related social needs provide a more granular understanding of the experience of social risk factors at a particular moment. These are self-reported and center individual and family preferences in the prioritization of social care. Using the housing stability example, we recognize that a family may indeed be experiencing (and report) housing instability as a social risk factor but may choose to decline assistance addressing that risk factor because of their understanding and prioritization of time and resources. In this example, we can say that this family is experiencing a social risk factor but not an HRSN. This distinction brings the shared decision-making model into social care, defining a risk as an HRSN only if a patient or family requests assistance with that need. As the literature supports,[18,19] there are often discrepancies between those reporting social risks and those reporting HRSNs, so this distinction in terminology is important in identifying those suitable for and amenable to assistance activities.

Key Concept

Under the umbrella term of *social determinants of health,* specific nomenclature allows for further distinctions in our understanding of how health is socially determined.

Structural determinants of health: **The socioeconomic and political mechanisms at the community level that generate inequities in the social causes of health.**

Social causes of health: **The material circumstances and behavioral, biological, and psychosocial factors influencing health outcomes for all individuals. These can be either social assets (positive) or social risks (negative).**

Social risk factors: **Adverse, measurable individual-level socioeconomic conditions that influence individual health outcomes.**

Health-related social needs: **Adverse, self-reported individual-level social risk factors for which patients have expressed their preference for assistance.**

Structural Determinants of Health

Moving upstream from the individual experiences of social risk, we know that not all communities or individuals experience the social causes of health equally. The underlying processes that have shaped this unequal distribution have led to persistent inequities in health outcomes. Interventions that focus on the intermediary determinants of health, such as providing food pantry resources to a patient with food insecurity, may support that individual and improve their health outcomes in the short term; however, this intervention would fail to address the mechanisms that have systematically created inequities in the distribution of social causes of health among populations. Making sense of how these inequities have persisted, and for whom, requires understanding the intersection between the social, political, and cultural *context* and the socioeconomic *position* of individuals and families (the underlying structural determinants of health) that are laid out in **Figure 2-1**.

The context for the structural determinants of health includes social systems, political systems, and cultural systems, all of which are dynamic and embedded within institutions. Social systems that serve to perpetuate gradations of material resources include the education system, labor markets, and the criminal legal system. Political systems play a role as well, as they determine the structure of the state as it relates to redistributive and welfare policies. The cultural institutions of racism and caste underlie all aspects of this context.[20]

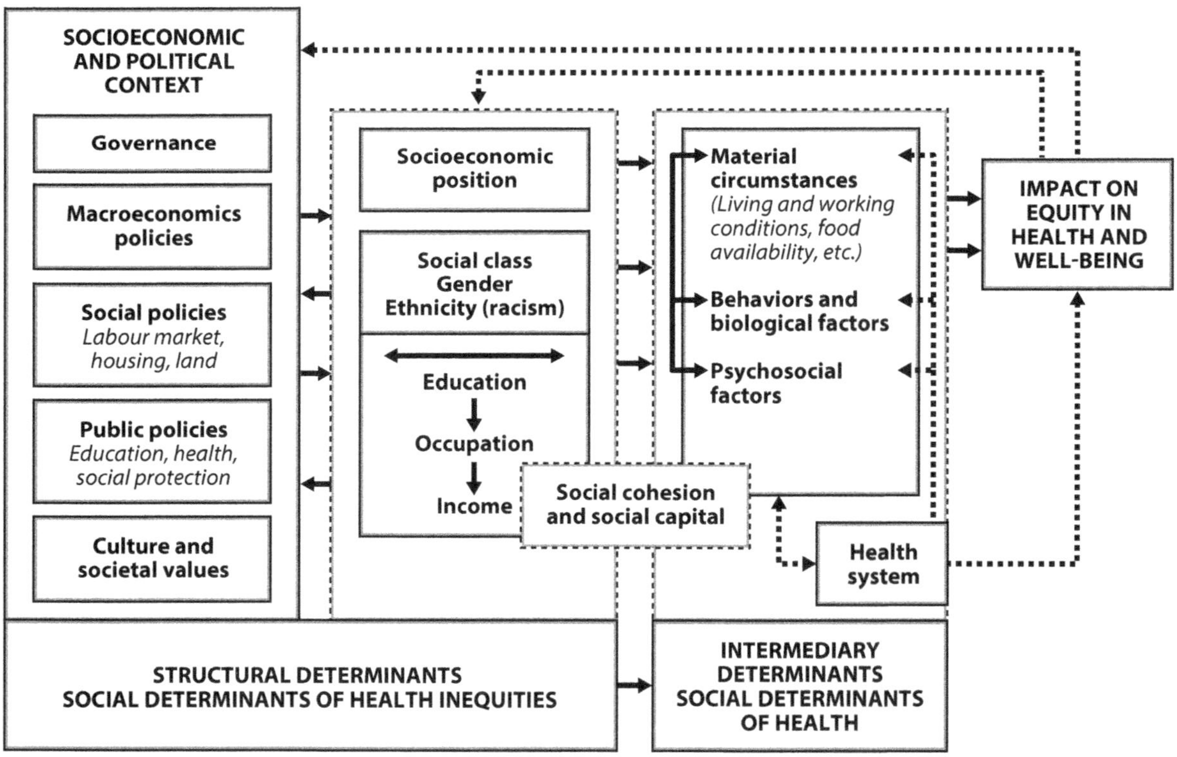

Figure 2-1. World Health Organization Committee on Social Determinants of Health Conceptual Framework

From Solar O, Irwin A. *A Conceptual Framework for Action on the Social Determinants of Health: Social Determinants of Health Discussion Paper 2 (Policy and Practice)*. World Health Organization; 2010:46. Accessed September 11, 2024. https://www.who.int/publications/i/item/9789241500852.

Social identities are important to understand in an intersectional framework, by acknowledging that most individuals inhabit multiple social identities (eg, race, class, gender), which interact to create new experiences of privilege or marginalization.[21] Often broad contextual factors then affect individuals by intersecting with these social identities, creating stratifications and social class divisions that define socioeconomic positions within hierarchies of power. In this way, the intersection of *context* and socioeconomic *position* determines individuals' places within social hierarchies.[22] These gradations of inequities in society then determine the distribution of social causes of health and the differential experiences of exposure and vulnerability.

For clinicians, understanding the HRSNs of individuals or families requires examining the contextual factors that have led to those needs, specifically the ways in which structural determinants of health have played out individually. As illustrated in **Figure 2-2**, the stream metaphor is often used to visually represent where clinical care sits in the ecosystem of determinants of health. Our role in clinical practice is downstream of the many SDOH, with screening for and addressing HRSNs sitting just upstream from clinical care. The distribution of HRSNs, however, is determined by the further-upstream structural determinants of health within communities.[23]

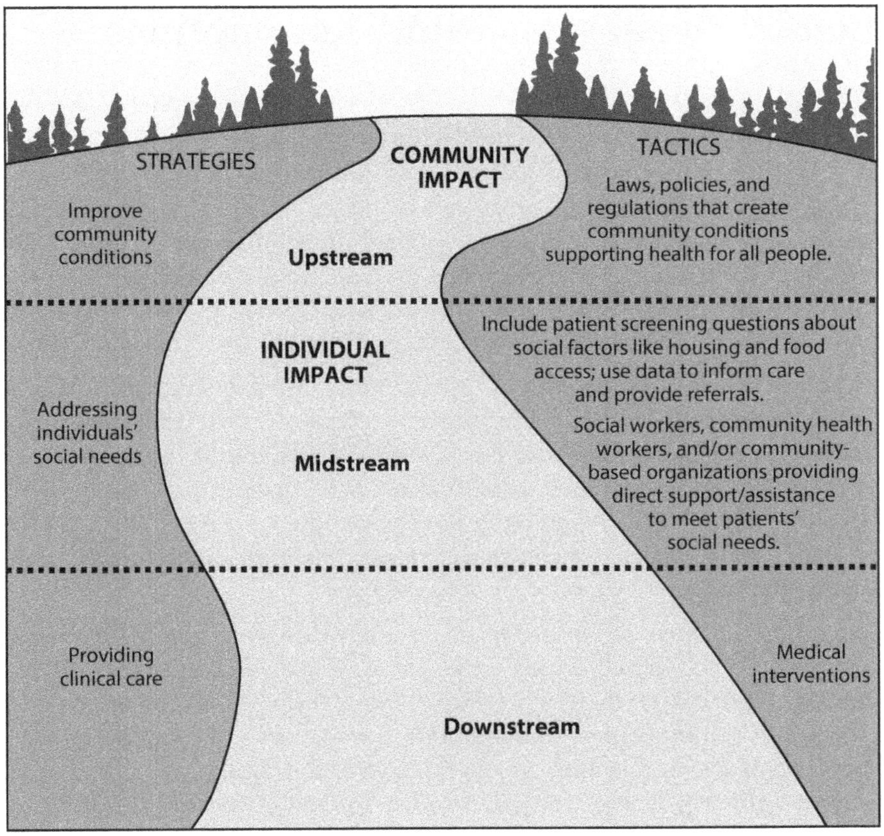

Figure 2-2. Stream Metaphor to Address Both Social and Structural Determinants of Health

Reproduced with permission from Castrucci B, Auerbach J. Meeting individual social needs falls short of addressing social determinants of health. *Health Affairs Forefront* blog. January 16, 2019. Accessed April 10, 2024. https://www.healthaffairs.org/content/forefront/meeting-individual-social-needs-falls-short-addressing-social-determinants-health.

Designing interventions to address downstream needs, then, requires intersectoral policies, addressing not only the intermediary determinants of health but also the upstream structural determinants that have produced the inequitable distribution of the intermediary determinants across communities.

Key Concept

Upstream systems (social, political, and cultural) create the context for inequities within society. The intersection of this context with individual identities (eg, race, class, gender) creates social hierarchies and an inequitable distribution of midstream (intermediary) determinants of health. Interventions to address health disparities must consider these upstream determinants in their design and evaluation.

Conceptual Challenges and Faulty Assumptions

Despite the growing clarity around frameworks and nomenclature for understanding the SDOH, there are some common underlying challenges and pitfalls for clinicians, researchers, and other health care professionals.[20]

First, the idea that individual causes of health can be added together to a sum of 100% has been a persistent reductionist fallacy.[24] Just as we know that not a single factor alone will influence a health outcome, individual interventions focusing on a single SDOH cannot be expected to have only direct effects on an outcome. Accounting for indirect effects, interaction effects, and multicausality often blurs the neat lines we as scientists try to draw between cause and effect.

Another important concept to understand as one embarks on work addressing the SDOH is linearity, specifically the assumption that determinants of health can be applied linearly to influence health outcomes. A greater number of identified HRSNs, for example, does not always lead to worse health outcomes in a linear fashion, as different social needs may play more or less prominent roles. Similarly, it is often challenging, if not impossible, to see predictable dose effects of social care interventions on health outcomes (ie, greater exposure to an intervention will lead to greater predictable improvement in a health outcome).

Finally, understanding the ways in which SDOH operate within hierarchies of power and access to resources is critical to contextualize this understanding. As we can see in the WHO conceptual framework (refer to **Figure 2-1**), there are clear feedback loops and bidirectional relationships between SDOH and health outcomes, so debunking the narrative of a unidirectional analysis (cause-and-effect pathways) is essential. As others have noted, health outcomes can be outcomes influenced by unmet HRSNs, as well as predictive variables that may worsen HRSNs.[25]

For clinicians sitting with individual patients, keeping these challenges in mind is important to ground the theoretical framing of these determinants of health. For researchers and scientists designing social care integration programs and evaluations, novel systems science approaches have been proposed that allow researchers to account for these challenges and build models that appropriately measure the complexity of these interactions.[20,26] Contextualizing and interpreting data in partnership with patients and community members may help mitigate some of these challenges and allow for more effective interventions that focus on shared priorities.[27]

Key Concept

Complex relationships exist between the social causes of health and the health of individuals and communities. Caution is warranted when drawing conclusions from these relationships, with particular attention to avoiding reductionism, in which the whole likely equals more than the sum of its parts. Social causes of health also likely contribute to health outcomes in nonlinear and bidirectional ways, so measuring both dose effects and cause-and-effect pathways of interventions on health outcomes is challenging at best and incorrect at worst. Contextualizing social causes of health in partnership with patients and community is one strategy that may lead to improved understanding and more effective interventions.

Health-Related Social Needs Screening in Health Systems

Why Address Health-Related Social Needs in Health Care?

Despite the relatively downstream position of HRSNs in the cascade of determinants of health outcomes, a strong body of evidence exists linking HRSNs to adverse health outcomes. Studies have elucidated the various mechanisms that link HRSNs to adverse health outcomes, including through increased exposure to risk factors for chronic disease, higher likelihood of chronic stress, and reduced access to resources for patients with preexisting conditions, among others.[28,29] Evidence has shown that patients with HRSNs also experience higher health care expenditures and utilization,[30] including more emergency department visits,[31–33] more hospital admissions,[34,35] higher rates of hospital readmission,[36] and higher rates of missed outpatient appointments.[37,38] Clinical interventions that have integrated social care by addressing food security,[39] housing stability,[40–42] and legal assistance[43,44] have been shown to improve both health outcomes and expenditures.

Key Concept

Patients with HRSNs face a greater likelihood of experiencing chronic illnesses, poorer control of those chronic illnesses, and greater health care utilization and expenditures. Interventions addressing upstream HRSNs have been shown to improve health outcomes as well as health care costs.

Health System Experiences With Health-Related Social Needs Screening

In recent years, health systems have increasingly shared their experiences implementing HRSN interventions, which may provide insight on best practices used in real-world settings. One large urban academic medical center in New York implemented an adapted HRSN screening tool across a network of 18 ambulatory primary care practices.[45] This health system witnessed significant variation in adoption of the screening tool by both practices and clinicians, despite screening a meaningful percentage of active patients. Heterogeneity was partially explained by the flexibility allowed in determining whom to screen and when, with some practices intending to screen all patients annually and others prioritizing only new patients. Additionally, there were significantly higher rates of adoption at practices with community health workers who provided direct social service navigation and linkage to care.

Another HRSN screening and referral program in NYC defined key challenges, facilitators, and best practices for implementation.[46] It identified several challenges to implementation, including the integration of screening into clinical workflows, the burden on staff, screening fatigue for patients, health literacy of patients, and staff capacity for data entry. Meanwhile, facilitators included existing collaborations with external social service organizations and direct provision of social services internally. The best practices they identified included integrating screening into existing workflows, adapting the screening tool, promoting universal screening, developing referral resources, using technology and data systems, and allocating dedicated staff.

Several other studies have reported additional barriers to screening, including staff time needed to administer the screening tool,[47–49] lack of training on HRSNs, and lack of resources to address the unmet HRSNs when they are identified.[48,50–52] Despite these barriers, there is growing consensus around the importance of not only screening for HRSNs but also going further to implement social service linkage and navigation. Clinicians, researchers, and patients have all made the case that screening for HRSNs without connecting patients to resources to address those needs is both ineffective and unethical.[52–54]

Evidence Gaps in Health-Related Social Needs Screening in Health Systems

Many health systems have now developed HRSN screening tools and interventions in response to recommendations and reporting mandates from the Centers for Medicare & Medicaid Services,[55] The Joint Commission,[56] the National Committee for Quality Assurance,[57] and other regulatory agencies. Although we have witnessed a recent wave of *social prescribing* in health systems,[58] there are still gaps in our understanding of how individual clinicians and health systems should address the HRSNs of their patients. Gottlieb and others highlight these key evidence gaps in their commentary, "Advancing Social Prescribing with Implementation Science," in which they identify the need to understand the acceptability of screening, availability and effectiveness of screening tools, and adaptation of tools and interventions in real-world settings.[59] There is also a demonstrated need to better understand workforce models for social care interventions, including comparing the use of clinical staff (ie, nurses, clinicians) and nonclinical staff (ie, social workers, community health workers, student volunteers), identifying and standardizing training and certification for staff, and evaluating strategies for staff retention and career advancement. Additionally, innovative payment models (eg, Medicaid 1115 demonstrations, detailed in the 1115 Waiver section of Chapter 3, Guidelines and Policies for Integrating Social Care Into Clinical Practice) need to be studied further to determine which can support, incentivize, and sustain social-prescribing interventions, including the required staff and technology infrastructure.

Key Concept

Changes in regulatory policies on the federal and state levels are increasingly mandating the collection of HRSN data in clinical care environments. Linkages with incentive payments have begun to facilitate this, because a key pillar of the White House playbook[1] to address the SDOH includes marshaling flexible funding mechanisms to support these efforts.

Integration of Social Care Into Medical Care to Address the Social Determinants of Health

Health-related social needs screening and navigation are important critical steps for clinicians and health systems to take to begin addressing the intermediary determinants of health. As laid out in *The U.S. Playbook on Social Determinants of Health,*[1] expanding data gathering (HRSN screening) is one of the 3 important pillars of the strategy to address the SDOH. But these interventions are insufficient alone in the larger struggle to address the SDOH and health inequities. While the White House has identified funding priorities and supporting "community backbone organizations" as additional pillars in its playbook, health systems also wield tremendous power to influence the upstream context within which health inequities persist. This power can and should be brought to bear in designing and implementing multi-sectoral interventions to address the structural determinants of health as well as shift the distribution of social causes in ways that can fundamentally address health inequities.

Key Points

- The idea of health as socially determined is not a new concept; however, spending on social care programs in the United States has not grown in proportion to our growing understanding of its role in determining health outcomes.
- Intermediary SDOH, as defined by the WHO framework, includes the material circumstances and behavioral, biological, and social factors that influence health outcomes. These can act as either social assets (positive) or social risks (negative).
- Health-related social needs are adverse, self-reported individual-level socioeconomic risk factors for which patients have expressed their preference for assistance.
- The distribution of intermediary determinants of health (assets or risks) is inherently inequitable, influenced by the socioeconomic, political, and cultural *context* and the socioeconomic *position* of individuals and families (the structural determinants of health).
- Health-related social needs screening has recently gained traction within health systems. There is a strong evidence base supporting this work; however, large gaps remain in our understanding of the implementation challenges across complex health care delivery systems.
- To address the intermediary SDOH, screening for and addressing HRSNs is necessary for health systems.
- To reduce health inequities, interventions must move upstream, going beyond addressing HRSNs into requiring multi-sectoral policies and approaches.

References

1. Domestic Policy Council. *The U.S. Playbook to Address Social Determinants of Health*. White House Office of Science and Technology Policy; 2023
2. Waitzkin H. The social origins of illness: a neglected history. *Int J Health Serv*. 1981;11(1):77–103 PMID: 7016768 doi: 10.2190/5CDV-P4FE-Y6HN-JACD
3. Williams DR, Sternthal M. Understanding racial-ethnic disparities in health: sociological contributions. *J Health Soc Behav*. 2010;51(suppl):S15–S27 PMID: 20943580 doi: 10.1177/0022146510383838
4. Regional Office for Europe. *Declaration of Alma-Ata*. World Health Organization; 1978. Accessed July 3, 2024. https://iris.who.int/handle/10665/347879
5. World Health Organization. Social determinants of health. Accessed July 3, 2024. https://www.who.int/health-topics/social-determinants-of-health#tab=tab_1
6. Committee on Integrating Social Needs Care Into the Delivery of Health Care to Improve the Nation's Health. *Integrating Social Care Into the Delivery of Health Care: Moving Upstream to Improve the Nation's Health*. National Academies of Sciences, Engineering, and Medicine; 2019
7. Gitterman BA, Flanagan PJ, Cotton WH, et al; American Academy of Pediatrics Council on Community Pediatrics. Poverty and child health in the United States. *Pediatrics*. 2016;137(4):e20160339 PMID: 26962238 doi: 10.1542/peds.2016-0339
8. Papanicolas I, Woskie LR, Jha AK. Health care spending in the United States and other high-income countries. *JAMA*. 2018;319(10):1024–1039 PMID: 29536101 doi: 10.1001/jama.2018.1150
9. Papanicolas I, Woskie LR, Orlander D, Orav EJ, Jha AK. The relationship between health spending and social spending in high-income countries: how does the US compare? *Health Aff (Millwood)*. 2019;38(9):1567–1575 PMID: 31411912 doi: 10.1377/hlthaff.2018.05187
10. Bradley EH, Canavan M, Rogan E, et al. Variation in health outcomes: the role of spending on social services, public health, and health care, 2000–09. *Health Aff (Millwood)*. 2016;35(5):760–768 PMID: 27140980 doi: 10.1377/hlthaff.2015.0814
11. Tikkanen RS, Schneider EC. Social spending to improve population health—does the United States spend as wisely as other countries? *N Engl J Med*. 2020;382(10):885–887 PMID: 32130810 doi: 10.1056/NEJMp1916585
12. Racine AD. Child poverty and the health care system. *Acad Pediatr*. 2016;16(3)(suppl):S83–S89 PMID: 27044708 doi: 10.1016/j.acap.2015.12.002
13. Currie J. What we say and what we do: why US investments in children's health are falling short. *Health Aff (Millwood)*. 2020;39(10):1684–1692 PMID: 33017250 doi: 10.1377/hlthaff.2020.00633
14. Solar O, Irwin A. *A Conceptual Framework for Action on the Social Determinants of Health: Social Determinants of Health Discussion Paper 2 (Debates, Policy & Practice, Case Studies)*. World Health Organization; 2010. Accessed September 11, 2024. https://www.who.int/publications/i/item/9789241500852
15. Alderwick H, Gottlieb LM. Meanings and misunderstandings: a social determinants of health lexicon for health care systems. *Milbank Q*. 2019;97(2):407–419 PMID: 31069864 doi: 10.1111/1468-0009.12390
16. Eder M, Henninger M, Durbin S, et al. Screening and interventions for social risk factors: technical brief to support the US Preventive Services Task Force. *JAMA*. 2021;326(14):1416–1428 PMID: 34468710 doi: 10.1001/jama.2021.12825
17. Frederick TJ, Chwalek M, Hughes J, Karabanow J, Kidd S. How stable is stable? defining and measuring housing stability. *J Community Psychol*. 2014;42(8):964–979 doi: 10.1002/jcop.21665
18. Bottino CJ, Rhodes ET, Kreatsoulas C, Cox JE, Fleegler EW. Food insecurity screening in pediatric primary care: can offering referrals help identify families in need? *Acad Pediatr*. 2017;17(5):497–503 PMID: 28302365 doi: 10.1016/j.acap.2016.10.006

19. Schiavoni KH, Helscel K, Vogeli C, et al. Prevalence of social risk factors and social needs in a Medicaid accountable care organization (ACO). *BMC Health Serv Res.* 2022;22(1):1375 PMID: 36403024 doi: 10.1186/s12913-022-08721-9

20. Jayasinghe S. Social determinants of health inequalities: towards a theoretical perspective using systems science. *Int J Equity Health.* 2015;14(1):71 PMID: 26303914 doi: 10.1186/s12939-015-0205-8

21. Crenshaw K. Mapping the margins: intersectionality, identity politics, and violence against women of color. *Stanford Law Rev.* 1991;43(6):1241–1299 doi: 10.2307/1229039

22. Wilson Y, White A, Jefferson A, Danis M. Intersectionality in clinical medicine: the need for a conceptual framework. *Am J Bioeth.* 2019;19(2):8–19 PMID: 30784384 doi: 10.1080/15265161.2018.1557275

23. Castrucci B, Auerbach J. Meeting individual social needs falls short of addressing social determinants of health. *Health Affairs Forefront* blog. January 16, 2019. Accessed April 10, 2024. https://www.healthaffairs.org/content/forefront/meeting-individual-social-needs-falls-short-addressing-social-determinants-health

24. Krieger N. Health equity and the fallacy of treating causes of population health as if they sum to 100. *Am J Public Health.* 2017;107(4):541–549 PMID: 28272952 doi: 10.2105/ajph.2017.303655

25. McQueen A, Roberts C, Garg R, et al. Specialized tobacco quitline and basic needs navigation interventions to increase cessation among low income smokers: study protocol for a randomized controlled trial. *Contemp Clin Trials.* 2019;80:40–47 PMID: 30904596 doi: 10.1016/j.cct.2019.03.009

26. Fink DS, Keyes KM, Cerdá M. Social determinants of population health: a systems sciences approach. *Curr Epidemiol Rep.* 2016;3(1):98–105 PMID: 27642548 doi: 10.1007/s40471-016-0066-8

27. Cashman SB, Adeky S, Allen AJ III, et al. The power and the promise: working with communities to analyze data, interpret findings, and get to outcomes. *Am J Public Health.* 2008;98(8):1407–1417 PMID: 18556617 doi: 10.2105/AJPH.2007.113571

28. Heller CG, Rehm CD, Parsons AH, Chambers EC, Hollingsworth NH, Fiori KP. The association between social needs and chronic conditions in a large, urban primary care population. *Prev Med.* 2021;153:106752 PMID: 34348133 doi: 10.1016/j.ypmed.2021.106752

29. Green KA, Bovell-Ammon A, Sandel M. Housing and neighborhoods as root causes of child poverty. *Acad Pediatr.* 2021;21(8)(suppl):S194–S199 PMID: 34740428 doi: 10.1016/j.acap.2021.08.018

30. Bensken WP, Alberti PM, Stange KC, Sajatovic M, Koroukian SM. ICD-10 Z-code health-related social needs and increased healthcare utilization. *Am J Prev Med.* 2022;62(4):e232–e241 PMID: 34865935 doi: 10.1016/j.amepre.2021.10.004

31. Jones KG, Roth SE, Vartanian KB. Health and health care use strongly associated with cumulative burden of social determinants of health. *Popul Health Manag.* 2022;25(2):218–226 PMID: 34935504 doi: 10.1089/pop.2021.0255

32. Holcomb J, Highfield L, Ferguson GM, Morgan RO. Association of social needs and healthcare utilization among Medicare and Medicaid beneficiaries in the Accountable Health Communities Model. *J Gen Intern Med.* 2022;37(14):3692–3699 PMID: 35132551 doi: 10.1007/s11606-022-07403-w

33. Davis CI, Montgomery AE, Dichter ME, Taylor LD, Blosnich JR. Social determinants and emergency department utilization: findings from the Veterans Health Administration. *Am J Emerg Med.* 2020;38(9):1904–1909 PMID: 32739860 doi: 10.1016/j.ajem.2020.05.078

34. Conroy K, Samnaliev M, Cheek S, Chien AT. Pediatric primary care–based social needs services and health care utilization. *Acad Pediatr.* 2021;21(8):1331–1337 PMID: 33516898 doi: 10.1016/j.acap.2021.01.012

35. Wurster Ovalle VM, Beck AF, Ollberding NJ, Klein MD. Social risk screening in pediatric primary care anticipates acute care utilization. *Pediatr Emerg Care.* 2021;37(10):e609–e614 PMID: 32149994 doi: 10.1097/PEC.0000000000001979

36. McQueen A, Li L, Herrick CJ, et al. Social needs, chronic conditions, and health care utilization among Medicaid beneficiaries. *Popul Health Manag*. 2021;24(6):681–690 PMID: 33989068 doi: 10.1089/pop.2021.0065

37. Fiori KP, Heller CG, Rehm CD, et al. Unmet social needs and no-show visits in primary care in a US northeastern urban health system, 2018–2019. *Am J Public Health*. 2020;110(suppl 2):S242–S250 PMID: 32663075 doi: 10.2105/AJPH.2020.305717

38. Soto Mas F, Iriart C, Pedroncelli R, et al. Impact of health care and socioeconomic needs on health care utilization and disease management: the University of New Mexico Hospital Care One Program. *Popul Health Manag*. 2019;22(2):113–119 PMID: 29969375 doi: 10.1089/pop.2018.0048

39. Berkowitz SA, Terranova J, Hill C, et al. Meal delivery programs reduce the use of costly health care in dually eligible Medicare and Medicaid beneficiaries. *Health Aff (Millwood)*. 2018;37(4):535–542 PMID: 29608345 doi: 10.1377/hlthaff.2017.0999

40. Nelson RE, Montgomery AE, Suo Y, et al. Temporary financial assistance decreased health care costs for veterans experiencing housing instability. *Health Aff (Millwood)*. 2021;40(5):820–828 PMID: 33939508 doi: 10.1377/hlthaff.2020.01796

41. Wright BJ, Vartanian KB, Li HF, Royal N, Matson JK. Formerly homeless people had lower overall health care expenditures after moving into supportive housing. *Health Aff (Millwood)*. 2016;35(1):20–27 PMID: 26733697 doi: 10.1377/hlthaff.2015.0393

42. Bovell-Ammon A, Mansilla C, Poblacion A, et al. Housing intervention for medically complex families associated with improved family health: pilot randomized trial. *Health Aff (Millwood)*. 2020;39(4):613–621 PMID: 32250672 doi: 10.1377/hlthaff.2019.01569

43. Beck AF, Henize AW, Qiu T, et al. Reductions in hospitalizations among children referred to a primary care–based medical-legal partnership. *Health Aff (Millwood)*. 2022;41(3):341–349 PMID: 35254924 doi: 10.1377/hlthaff.2021.00905

44. Yan AF, Chen Z, Wang Y, et al. Effectiveness of social needs screening and interventions in clinical settings on utilization, cost, and clinical outcomes: a systematic review. *Health Equity*. 2022;6(1):454–475 PMID: 35801145 doi: 10.1089/heq.2022.0010

45. Fiori KP, Heller CG, Flattau A, et al. Scaling-up social needs screening in practice: a retrospective, cross-sectional analysis of data from electronic health records from Bronx county, New York, USA. *BMJ Open*. 2021;11(9):e053633 PMID: 34588265 doi: 10.1136/bmjopen-2021-053633

46. Berry C, Paul M, Massar R, Marcello RK, Krauskopf M. Social needs screening and referral program at a large US public hospital system, 2017. *Am J Public Health*. 2020;110(suppl 2):S211–S214 PMID: 32663088 doi: 10.2105/AJPH.2020.305642

47. Kostelanetz S, Pettapiece-Phillips M, Weems J, et al. Health care professionals' perspectives on universal screening of social determinants of health: a mixed-methods study. *Popul Health Manag*. 2022;25(3):367–374 PMID: 34698559 doi: 10.1089/pop.2021.0176

48. Schickedanz A, Hamity C, Rogers A, Sharp AL, Jackson A. Clinician experiences and attitudes regarding screening for social determinants of health in a large integrated health system. *Med Care*. 2019;57(6)(suppl 2):S197–S201 PMID: 31095061 doi: 10.1097/MLR.0000000000001051

49. Brown J, Ahmed N, Biel M, et al. Considerations in implementation of social risk factor screening and referral in maternal and infant care in Washington, DC: a qualitative study. *PLoS One*. 2023;18(4):e0283815 PMID: 37053233 doi: 10.1371/journal.pone.0283815

50. Tong ST, Liaw WR, Kashiri PL, et al. Clinician experiences with screening for social needs in primary care. *J Am Board Fam Med*. 2018;31(3):351–363 PMID: 29743219 doi: 10.3122/jabfm.2018.03.170419

51. Jackson CL, Hood E, Jenkins JA, Szanton SL. Barriers and facilitators to nurses addressing social needs and associated outcomes in the ambulatory setting in adult patients: systematic review. *J Adv Nurs*. 2023;79(7):2444–2455 PMID: 37073871 doi: 10.1111/jan.15670

52. Hamity C, Jackson A, Peralta L, Bellows J. Perceptions and experience of patients, staff, and clinicians with social needs assessment. *Perm J.* 2018;22:18–105 PMID: 30285914 doi: 10.7812/TPP/18-105
53. Hare AJ, Honig K, Cronholm PF, Shabazz-McKlaine S, Morgan AU. Patient perspectives on technology-based approaches to social needs screening. *Am J Manag Care.* 2023;29(1):e18–e23 PMID: 36716160 doi: 10.37765/ajmc.2023.89309
54. Garg A, Boynton-Jarrett R, Dworkin PH. Avoiding the unintended consequences of screening for social determinants of health. *JAMA.* 2016;316(8):813–814 PMID: 27367226 doi: 10.1001/jama.2016.9282
55. CMS Office of Minority Health. *CMS Framework for Health Equity 2022–2032.* Centers for Medicare & Medicaid Services; 2022. Accessed April 25, 2024. https://www.cms.gov/priorities/health-equity/minority-health/equity-programs/framework
56. Joint Commission. New requirements to reduce health care disparities. *R3 Rep.* 2022;36
57. *Social Determinants of Health Resource Guide.* National Committee for Quality Assurance; 2020. NCQA publication 1181-0720
58. Oster C, Skelton C, Leibbrandt R, Hines S, Bonevski B. Models of social prescribing to address non-medical needs in adults: a scoping review. *BMC Health Serv Res.* 2023;23(1):642 PMID: 37316920 doi: 10.1186/s12913-023-09650-x
59. Gottlieb L, Cottrell EK, Park B, Clark KD, Gold R, Fichtenberg C. Advancing social prescribing with implementation science. *J Am Board Fam Med.* 2018;31(3):315–321 PMID: 29743213 doi: 10.3122/jabfm.2018.03.170249

CHAPTER 3

Guidelines and Policies for Integrating Social Care Into Clinical Practice

Milani Patel, MD, FAAP

Health-related social needs (HRSNs) influence downstream health outcomes. This recognition is transforming clinical practice across all settings. Professional health care organizations have issued policy statements over the past 10 years, delineating the importance of recognizing and screening for HRSNs. These guidelines also include recommendations for how policymakers and health systems can address these social needs. Over the same period, federal and state entities have collaborated in proposing financing mechanisms to incentivize programming to address social drivers of health (also referred to as *social determinants of health*).

CHAPTER 3

Guidelines and Policies for Integrating Social Care Into Clinical Practice

Milani Patel, MD, FAAP

Introduction

Health-related social needs (HRSNs), such as food insecurity and transportation barriers, can significantly affect the health and well-being of patients. Health care organizations and the social care sector must align in care coordination if we are to address these needs and have a measurable impact on downstream health outcomes. This recognition has evolved over the past decade in various health care settings and is reflected in the guidance of national professional health care organizations. These recommendations vary depending on the field of medicine, but commonalities include systematic screening, a team-based approach to incorporating HRSN processes into the clinical setting, and community resource collaboration to address these needs. On a broader scale, professional organizations also acknowledge the need for increased governmental funding for social needs–related programming and enhanced payment models to incentivize screening and subsequent interventions for unmet HRSNs. Governmental agencies, including the Centers for Medicare & Medicaid Services (CMS), have introduced financing for HRSN programming at the state level.

Evidence for Social Drivers of Health–Related Guidelines and Policies

Poverty influences the environment in which a child is born and raised, leading to adverse circumstances that negatively affect their health (eg, low birth weight, increased infant mortality, speech delay, high risk for chronic illness, poor nutrition, and high likelihood of injury).[1] The stress of poverty may also influence parenting style, as factors such as food and housing insecurities can lead to poorer parenting, which results in children lacking adequate support and having difficulties with self-regulation, inattention, impulsivity, and peer relationships.[2] Poverty causes toxic stress, defined as the "excessive or prolonged activation of the physiologic stress response systems in the absence of the buffering protection afforded by stable, responsive relationships."[3] Toxic stress has been shown to alter genomic function and lead to neuroendocrine dysregulation, which affects the way the brain functions. Toxic stress can contribute to chronic cardiovascular, immune, and psychiatric conditions.[4] The vicious cycle of poverty has been clearly demonstrated, continuing from one generation to the next. For example, poverty can make it difficult to graduate high school. Adolescents who do not graduate high school are more likely to experience adolescent parenthood, unsteady jobs, or incarceration.[5] Among highly industrialized countries, the United States ranks the lowest in social mobility.[6]

Screening for HRSNs is the first step in identifying the factors that can influence health outcomes for children later in life. Road maps can then be developed to address elicited needs for true social care integration. Examples include expanding the workforce to include a social care staff, streamlining a referral process to community organizations, or optimizing existing resources in the health care setting to meet these needs. In response to the extensive literature on the nature of poverty on child health, various pediatric-related professional organizations and publications have focused on the importance of screening for and addressing HRSNs and have published guidance for clinical teams.

Key Concept

Poverty and HRSNs that stem from poverty may cause toxic stress, which has been shown to contribute to chronic medical conditions later in life. Screening for and addressing HRSNs can mitigate the effects of toxic stress.

Professional Health Care Organization Policy Statements

Since 2016, various professional health care organizations have issued policy statements (discussed here in chronological order) defining and addressing the social drivers of health (SDOH), as well as specific action items pertinent to their field.

American Academy of Pediatrics

The American Academy of Pediatrics (AAP) published its policy statement "Poverty and Child Health in the United States" in 2016, building on previous AAP policies on child health equity, housing insecurity, and early childhood adversity.[7] Importantly, the policy highlights that "the early detection of poverty-related disorders is an important and emerging component of pediatric scope of practice."

First and foremost, the policy emphasizes the importance of a family-centered medical home to assess the financial stability of families and link them to community resources. It outlines how clinical teams can transform their practice into one that recognizes the importance of HRSNs. Educating all members of the health care team (eg, front desk staff, nurses, billing, clinicians) on HRSNs is essential so families are viewed through a lens of understanding that numerous factors may act as barriers to parents seeking health care for their child, such as work schedules and transportation challenges. Rather than simply deny care for a patient who is late to their appointment, through a family-centered lens, the front desk staff member might elicit that the parent had been waiting for a delayed city bus and offer the family an opportunity to wait to be seen as the pediatrician's schedule permits.

Screening for HRSNs in clinical practice with health care staff or paper/tablet-based self-administered questionnaires is essential in detecting social needs and is explored further in Chapter 4, Screening for Social Needs in the Pediatric Clinical Setting. Likewise, eliciting resilience and protective factors is important. By approaching families from a strengths-based perspective, health care professionals can build trust and rapport and identify assets that can help ameliorate the sequelae of financial insecurity and poverty.

The AAP policy statement summarizes governmental programs that exist to directly address financial insecurity among families, such as Earned Income Tax Credit (EITC); Child Tax Credit; Temporary Assistance for Needy Families (TANF); Special Supplemental Nutrition Program for Women, Infants, and Children (WIC); Supplemental Nutrition Assistance Program (SNAP); and the National School Lunch Program, all of which will be discussed in further depth in Chapters 5, Financial Assistance and Access to Care, and 7, Food Insecurity. The policy statement also proposes coordinating with existing parenting and literacy programs to facilitate referrals, such as Head Start (www.acf.hhs.gov/ohs), HealthySteps (www.healthysteps.org), Triple P (https://triplep-parenting.com), and Reach Out and Read (https://reachoutandread.org). Health care professionals should try to acquaint themselves with local community resources, such as local libraries, medical-legal partnerships, food banks, home visiting programs, and local health departments, and then build relationships with them. To learn more about food banks, refer to the Food Banks section of Chapter 7, Food Insecurity.

Finally, beyond individual support and community resources, the AAP policy statement highlights the value of advocating for policy change at local, state, and federal levels, based on research outcomes from rigorous studies and analyses. The policy asks health care professionals to engage in advocacy for funding toward the following activities: quality early childhood programs, which have shown significant financial return on early investments; financial benefit programs such as WIC and SNAP; home visiting programs; job training opportunities; affordable housing; enhanced medical-home services such as care coordination and mental health treatment; and school-readiness and parenting-support initiatives.

Bright Futures

Bright Futures is a national health promotion and prevention initiative, led by the AAP and supported by the US Department of Health and Human Services and the Maternal and Child Health Bureau.[8] Using a strengths-based approach, it provides theory-based and evidence-driven guidelines for all preventive care screenings, such as lead screening, and for 31 health supervision visits at established intervals based on age. It has been widely adopted as the standard of care for children, adolescents, and young adults through age 21 years and is revised every few years.

The fourth edition, published in 2017, includes special emphasis on the SDOH as an area of "vital importance to caring for children and families" and encourages health care professionals to ask about topics at each health supervision visit such as food insecurity, domestic violence, substance use, housing situations, and other issues that may affect a family's health. Bright Futures is recognized as the standard for pediatric preventive health insurance coverage and has been adopted by numerous state Medicaid plans, more of which is discussed in the Financing Approaches to Support Health-Related Social Needs section later in this chapter.

Academic Pediatric Association

The Academic Pediatric Association (APA) Childhood Poverty Task Force Health Care Delivery Committee published an evidence-based, practical approach to screening for HRSNs in 2016 entitled "Screening for Social Determinants of Health Among Children and Families Living in Poverty: A Guide for Clinicians," recognizing that although health care professionals are in a unique position to prevent adversity by screening for social needs, they need concrete tools and resources to effectively do so.[9]

Screening and surveillance, over the course of multiple health supervision visits, should prioritize identified areas of need that exist within that community and should ideally be implemented only after resources are identified. Screening can be done with a single tool by using a team-based approach. Screening does not necessarily need to fall on the health care professional but can be completed by a nonphysician staff member. Screening should be universal among patients to decrease stigma. The APA guidelines provide a comprehensive summary of the following HRSNs: child maltreatment, child care and education, family financial support, physical environment, family social support, intimate partner violence, maternal/birthing parent depression and family mental illness, household substance use, firearm exposure, and parental health literacy. To serve as a practical resource, the guidelines also use easy-to-navigate tables to outline and link to available screening tools and existing resources for each HRSN.

Key Concept

The AAP and APA recommend a team-based approach to screening for HRSNs and linkage to local community resources. The AAP encourages active participation in advocacy efforts to increase governmental funding toward social programs.

American College of Physicians

The Health and Public Policy Committee of the American College of Physicians (ACP) published a position paper in 2018 based on literature review, policy documents, and field expertise on the SDOH as they relate to the practice of internal medicine and its subspecialties.[10] After defining key nonmedical drivers of health, such as socioeconomic status, housing, transportation, food and agriculture, and information technology, they acknowledge the impact of SDOH on racial and ethnic health disparities. The statement goes on to outline federal and local government initiatives to address SDOH, such as Healthy People 2020, the Older Americans Act, grant programming through the CMS, and the Fruit and Vegetable Prescription Program. They conclude with action item recommendations to empower their constituents to advocate for health equity and the elimination of disparities. The first recommendation is the support of public policy interventions that address downstream socioeconomic inequalities. They emphasize that although individual interventions, such as opening more grocery stores in a "food desert," may seem consequential, it is public policy initiatives at the broader level that will have the most impact. They recommend the incorporation of SDOH teaching at all levels of medical education and mention how the Accreditation Council for Graduate Medical Education now audits residency programs for education on health care disparities. Third, they highlight the importance of a team-based collaboration approach in addressing SDOH, such as the Patient-Centered Medical Home model. Central to their recommendations is increased and more efficient funding for agencies that serves to reduce health disparities, as less than 10% of current health care expenditures in the United States are geared toward prevention and social services. Along the same lines is a call for support of large-scale research studies and community-based participatory research studies that evaluate outcomes of SDOH on populations with limited access to health care resources. The ACP also recommends health impact assessments to guide community planning activities to prevent triggers of negative social drivers. For example, in a "health in all policies" approach in 2014, tens of thousands of public schools became eligible for funding for the school breakfast and lunch programs for low-income families based on rates of participation in SNAP and TANF, rather than on paper applications, impacting millions of families. Optimal use of the electronic health record (EHR) is integral to collecting SDOH data and using these data to improve individual and community health, for example through Z codes to document social drivers for patients. The final recommendation is the support of quality payment models and performance measurement evaluations to recognize the increased risk of caring for populations who are disadvantaged because of limited financial and medical resources.

American College of Obstetricians and Gynecologists

The American College of Obstetricians and Gynecologists (ACOG) recognizes that HRSNs are associated with many conditions treated by obstetrician-gynecologists, such as preterm birth, unintended pregnancy, infertility, cervical cancer, breast cancer, and maternal mortality. In a committee opinion, "Importance of Social Determinants of Health and Cultural Awareness in the Delivery of Reproductive Health Care," released in 2018 and reaffirmed in 2021, the ACOG expands on the notion that health care decisions are not only an individual-level behavior but the result of systemic barriers that create and maintain inequalities.[11] It reflects on how discrimination, shared histories, and immigration status can all contribute to how a patient feels about and engages with the health care system. For example, a pregnant patient who is an undocumented immigrant may not seek out prenatal care for fear of deportation and may present to the emergency department (ED) only once in labor. A Black teenager may decline a long-acting reversible contraceptive out of fear caused by the history of experimentation on members of her race in the United States. Only by acknowledging these current and historical factors can we provide a truly patient-centered approach.

To this end, the ACOG recommends screening and documenting HRSNs, maximizing referrals to social service organizations, providing access to interpreter services at all levels of care, acknowledging that institutionalized racism serves as an SDOH, recognizing that stereotypes based on presumed cultural beliefs can negatively affect patient encounters, and advocating for policy changes that promote healthy living environments.

American Academy of Family Physicians

In 2018, the American Academy of Family Physicians (AAFP) published its position paper "Advancing Health Equity by Addressing the Social Determinants of Health in Family Medicine," focusing on the upstream macro-level factors (social, economic, and political mechanisms) that contribute to class inequalities.[12] These inequalities mediate living conditions, such as physical, social, economic, and work environments, that then mediate downstream factors such as risk behaviors, disease, injury, and mortality. For example, historical redlining, the practice of denying mortgages to certain racial populations, led to a lack of generational wealth among these groups. This can lead to financial insecurity a generation later, which can affect a child's nutrition, ultimately leading to obesity and a host of chronic illnesses in adulthood. The AAFP identified tangible steps physicians can take to address both upstream and downstream HRSNs, such as recognizing how HRSNs affect patients, addressing implicit bias in their practice, using cultural proficiency and health literacy standards, and advocating for public policies. The AAFP recognized the following public policies as important in reducing health inequities:

- Universal access to health care
- Health in all policies
- Federal nutrition programs

- Anti-poverty programs such as EITC
- Support for populations experiencing homelessness
- Antidiscrimination policies
- School funding to support educational achievement
- Built environment such as walkable neighborhoods
- Home visiting programs in early childhood
- Alternative payment models incorporating HRSNs
- Incorporation of HRSNs into medical education

Key Concept

In addition to screening for and addressing HRSNs, the ACP, ACOG, and AAFP further emphasize the role of systemic racism in HRSNs, the need for a social determinants curriculum at all levels of medical education, further research pertaining to HRSNs, and the need for alternative payment models.

National Academies of Science, Engineering, and Medicine

In 2019, the National Academies of Science, Engineering, and Medicine (NASEM) released its consensus study report "Integrating Social Care Into the Delivery of Health Care: Moving Upstream to Improve the Nation's Health."[13] The report was prompted by the increasing interest in the role of the health care sector in ameliorating social risk factors to achieve more equitable health outcomes. At the same time, there was a shift toward value-based payments that incentivized prevention and health care outcomes for populations instead of just health care service delivery. Together, these changes led to increased focus on upstream causes of poorer health outcomes. NASEM published its report in response to questions about how health care systems should address these HRSNs and what kind of infrastructure is needed to support these activities.

The committee identified 5 activities, *awareness, adjustment, assistance, alignment, and advocacy,* that would require systems-level changes to successfully implement. *Awareness* includes activities that identify social risks and strengths. For example, if a patient has no access to transportation in a city with poor public transportation options, *awareness* may include screening for transportation barriers via an EHR prompt. *Adjustment* refers to altering the provision of care to accommodate that barrier, such as offering a telehealth visit. *Assistance* means the connection of patients to social needs resources, such as arranging transport through Medicaid benefits. *Alignment* refers to activities undertaken by the health care system to understand what assets are available in the community and collaborate with those assets' contributors to positively influence health outcomes. In this case, it might be investing in a clinic shuttle to take patients to the closest bus stop. Finally, *advocacy* means partnering with other social care organizations to promote better policies, such as working with the city government on better public transportation options. The key necessities that would be required to implement these 5 activities include

- Adequately staffed and trained workforce
- Health information technology innovations
- New financing models

Regarding the workforce, the NASEM report acknowledges that all members of the interprofessional health team may have a role to play in carrying out these 5 activities, including physicians, nurses, aides, and volunteers. It is noted, however, that experts in social care, such as social workers and community health workers, should be specifically included in the workforce to effectively integrate social care into health care delivery and that federal, state, and institutional barriers should be addressed in ensuring that these workers are operating within the full scope of their practice and are being adequately compensated.

The NASEM committee found that the digitization of health care, spurred by financing from the federal government, far exceeds the monetary resources invested in the digitization of social care efforts. On a positive note, however, private equity has invested in health care start-ups that are working to address HRSNs. There are improvements to be made in data sharing between health care and social care organizations, although this needs to be balanced with data privacy and security. There is also a risk of exacerbating current health disparities by introducing technology, as all populations may not have access to the same technology.

Finally, financing for social care activities lags far behind financing for health care activities, when they should be viewed on a continuum. The cultural history of medicine is used as the basis of defining health care today and thus makes it less likely that social care will be included within that definition. Currently, within existing definitions of health care, state Medicaid plans and contracted managed health care plans are using a combination of amendments and waivers to meet social needs, which are described in the Financing Approaches to Support Health-Related Social Needs section further along in this chapter. There is great variation among states in the level of social care activity, as the CMS provides only limited guidance from a federal standpoint.

Given these findings, the NASEM committee recommended designing and financing health care delivery to include social care activities guided by awareness, adjustment, assistance, alignment, and advocacy; building a workforce to include social care in health care; developing a digital infrastructure to seamlessly communicate and share between health care and social care organizations; and conducting research to evaluate the efficacy of social care practices in health care settings.

Key Concept

The NASEM committee outlined systemic changes required by health care systems to build infrastructure that could meaningfully address HRSNs: awareness, adjustment, assistance, alignment, and advocacy.

These organizational guidelines from the AAP, APA, ACP, ACOG, AAFP, and NASEM (summarized in **Table 3-1**) outline the importance of investing in HRSNs to improve health outcomes for individuals and communities across the health care spectrum, reducing health care costs down the line. There has subsequently been greater interest in exploring and creating financing mechanisms for these initiatives, which we explore next. To address HRSNs, health care professionals and health systems may need to be resourceful and depend on nonmedical services or care in alternative settings, which may make reimbursement difficult.

Table 3-1. Summary of Health-Related Social Needs in Policy Statements by Professional Health Care Organizations

	AAP	Bright Futures	APA	ACP	ACOG	AAFP	NASEM
Social Needs Identified							
General discussion	X	X	X	X	X	X	X
Built environment	X		X			X	
Caregiver mental health		X	X				
Discrimination		X		X	X	X	
Early childhood development/child care	X	X	X			X	
Education	X	X	X			X	
Employment support	X						
Family violence		X	X				
Financial insecurity	X		X	X		X	
Firearm exposure		X	X				
Food insecurity	X	X	X	X		X	
Health literacy			X	X			
Housing		X	X	X		X	
Language barrier		X			X	X	
Medical insurance/access to care	X					X	
Parenting support	X					X	
Social supports		X	X				
Substance use		X	X				
Technology access				X			
Transportation				X	X		
Recommendations							
Community resource collaboration	X		X		X		X
Digital optimization				X			X
Enhanced payment models				X		X	X
Funding for HRSN research	X			X			X
Funding for specific social needs programs	X			X			
Health care professional education on HRSNs				X		X	X
"Health in all policies" approach				X	X	X	
Systematic HRSN screening	X		X	X	X		
Team-based approach				X			X

Abbreviations: AAFP, American Academy of Family Physicians; AAP, American Academy of Pediatrics; ACOG, American College of Obstetricians and Gynecologists; ACP, American College of Physicians; APA, Academic Pediatric Association; HRSN, health-related social need; NASEM, National Academy of Sciences, Engineering, and Medicine.

Financing Approaches to Support Health-Related Social Needs

General Medicaid Overview

In 1965, Medicaid became the first public health insurance program designed to serve the needs of US children living in low-income communities. Legislators soon added the Early and Periodic Screening, Diagnostic, and Treatment (EPSDT) benefit, outlining core preventive and diagnostic services pediatric patients should receive at their earliest point of need. These services are what we now recognize as the core elements (ie, hearing, vision, dental, immunizations) of pediatric health supervision visits.[14] Each state determines what is included as part of their EPSDT benefit. Often they consider AAP recommendations, specifically the Bright Futures periodicity schedule, as referenced in the Bright Futures section earlier in this chapter.[8] For instance, the AAP first recommended screening for maternal/birthing parent depression in 2008, and subsequently, many states covered it as a reimbursable service. As a result, more health care professionals started to incorporate parental depression screening as part of their practice. This response illustrates that the reimbursement of social care services by Medicaid could potentially serve as a key way to promote screening for HRSNs in the future. At present, Medicaid funds cannot directly be used to pay for nonmedical interventions. In recent years, however, the CMS has introduced strategies for state Medicaid plans to potentially address HRSNs, including in lieu of services benefits, the 1115 waiver, and alternative payment models.

In Lieu of Services Benefits

The term *in lieu of services* (ILOS) refers to payment for nonmedical services when medically appropriate and cost effective, such as a dehumidifier for a child with asthma or nutritious food for a child with diabetes. States can propose an ILOS that has been shown to be cost effective, through either a pilot program or existing literature. States who propose an ILOS and are granted approval, however, must prove that the services help prevent costly medical care down the line for a subsection of the population.[15] For example, California's CalAIM program began to offer nonmedical ILOS benefits in 2022, including housing transition navigation services, housing deposits, asthma remediation, and medically tailored meals. As of July 2023, the California Department of Health Care Services determined that these community supports were cost effective and, therefore, that further assessments of cost are no longer necessary.[16]

The 1115 Waiver

The 1115 waiver, also known as an 1115 demonstration, allows for more flexibility than ILOS and can be used by a state that wants to make experimental changes to its Medicaid program to address HRSNs, if the proposal promotes the objectives of the Medicaid program. As of May 2024, 21 states have an 1115 waiver with HRSN provisions, with 16 states pending.[17] For example, North Carolina's Healthy Opportunities Pilot program, approved in 2018 and implemented in 2022, authorized $650 million in Medicaid funding for a 5-year pilot. It covers about 1% to 2% of total Medicaid enrollees in the state. Pilot services for enrollees identified as having high needs, such as infants born prematurely or children with uncontrolled chronic conditions such as asthma, include evidence-based nonmedical services, such as case management, to address specific social needs related to housing, food, transportation, and interpersonal safety.[18]

Another example is the Whole Person Care (WPC) program in California, which ran from 2016 to 2021. The WPC program resulted in 25 simultaneous programs across 26 counties, with each program choosing its own population of focus and offerings. Populations of focus included people who had unstable living arrangements, people who frequently visited the ED, and people who had mental health concerns. Services included housing, employment support, medical respite care, and substance use support.[19]

As of May 2024, Arkansas, Arizona, Oregon, and Massachusetts have obtained approval to cover or expand services that address HRSNs in populations with high needs. Arkansas' Life360 HOMEs initiative (approval date: November 2022; currently active) provides care coordination for individuals with mental illness or substance use disorder who live in rural areas of the state, pregnant women and people who are at high risk for long-term poverty, and young adults who are involved in the judicial or foster care system. Arizona (approval date: October 2022; implementation expected 2024) will focus on housing support for individuals experiencing homelessness or who are at risk for homelessness with a documented health need. Building on existing programs, Massachusetts (approval date: September 2022; implementation expected 2025) will offer HRSN support to individuals who meet health-related criteria as well as have specific risk factors. Oregon (approval date: September 2022; implementation expected 2024) is specifically focusing on assisting populations in transition, such as individuals at risk for or experiencing homelessness, youth involved with the child welfare system, and those recently incarcerated.[17]

Key Concept

In lieu of services benefits and the 1115 demonstration are 2 approaches through Medicaid that states are using to address enrollees' HRSNs, with ongoing assessments to measure downstream impact.

Alternative Payment Models

Under traditional fee-for-service payment models, separate payments are made for each service provided. Social needs programs are generally not considered medical services and are not reimbursed. Over the past several years, however, pilot models for alternative payment models (APMs) supported by the CMS have emerged as key drivers to direct funding toward mitigating effects of HRSNs, including accountable care organizations, accountable health communities, and the Integrated Care for Kids Model.

Accountable Care Organizations

One type of APM is an accountable care organization (ACO). If an organization can achieve savings by providing high-quality and low-cost care to a defined group, the organization can share in those savings. This payment structure incentivizes physicians to work together to improve the care of patients. First started with private insurers and Medicare, it has now been extended into Medicaid, which is the largest insurer of children in the United States. A handful of states have organized their Medicaid programs around the ACO model for care delivery and, importantly, have recognized HRSNs as a critical problem. As a result, these states are requiring Medicaid programs and ACOs to address social drivers such as housing instability, food security and nutrition, and access to reliable transportation, often through partnership with community-based organizations. For example, Minnesota's Integrated Health Partnerships have served 460,000 residents and saved more than $200 million in 4 years. They have reduced hospital admissions by 14% and ED visits by 7%.[20]

Accountable Health Communities

The Accountable Health Communities (AHC) Model combines ACO delivery system resources and assets with public health and community improvement resources to address the broader social and economic factors that affect population health. Whereas ACOs address population health from a health care perspective, AHCs address health from a community perspective through collaboration between multiple partner organizations sharing responsibility for navigating HRSNs.

The Center for Medicare & Medicaid Innovation (CMMI), under the CMS, was tasked with designing, implementing, and testing new health care payment models to address growing concerns about rising costs, quality of care, and inefficient spending. From 2017 to 2022, the CMMI funded a $157 million AHC grant to pilot 3 models to evaluate HRSNs. The grant money was used to fund entities known as bridge organizations to implement the AHC Model within communities across the country in collaboration with clinical sites, community providers, state Medicaid agencies, and other community stakeholders. Bridge organizations were predominantly health systems and hospitals but also included nonprofits, health information technology innovators, academic institutions, payers, and a public health agency.[21]

All bridge organizations and clinical partners used the AHC HRSN Screening Tool (www.cms.gov/priorities/innovation/files/worksheets/ahcm-screeningtool.pdf) to screen beneficiaries for food insecurity, housing instability, transportation problems, utility difficulties, and interpersonal violence, across various clinical settings and via different modalities. At least 35% of patients reported at least 1 HRSN. Of these patients, those who demonstrated a high rate of ED utilization were then connected to community organizations through monthly patient navigation calls. Although the model inspired innovative community alignment work, it proved to be difficult to track navigation and resolution outcomes.[22]

Integrated Care for Kids Model

Child-focused APMs have been limited, but the willingness of health care payers to use these new payment models for other populations and conditions is promising for the application of APMs to children and families' health, social, and developmental needs. The Integrated Care for Kids (InCK) Model (**Figure 3-1**) is an example of a child-focused APM, with states and health care professionals sharing the responsibility for cost and outcomes. The model is a "child-centered local service delivery and state payment model that aims to reduce expenditures and improve quality of care for children...[through] prevention, early identification, and treatment of behavioral and physical health needs."[23] Primary goals of the InCK Model are to improve child health, reduce preventable inpatient stays, reduce out-of-home placements such as foster care, and create sustainable APMs. Funding for the model provides support for states and health care professionals to conduct early identification and treatment of children with health-related needs across settings. These needs include food and housing insecurity.

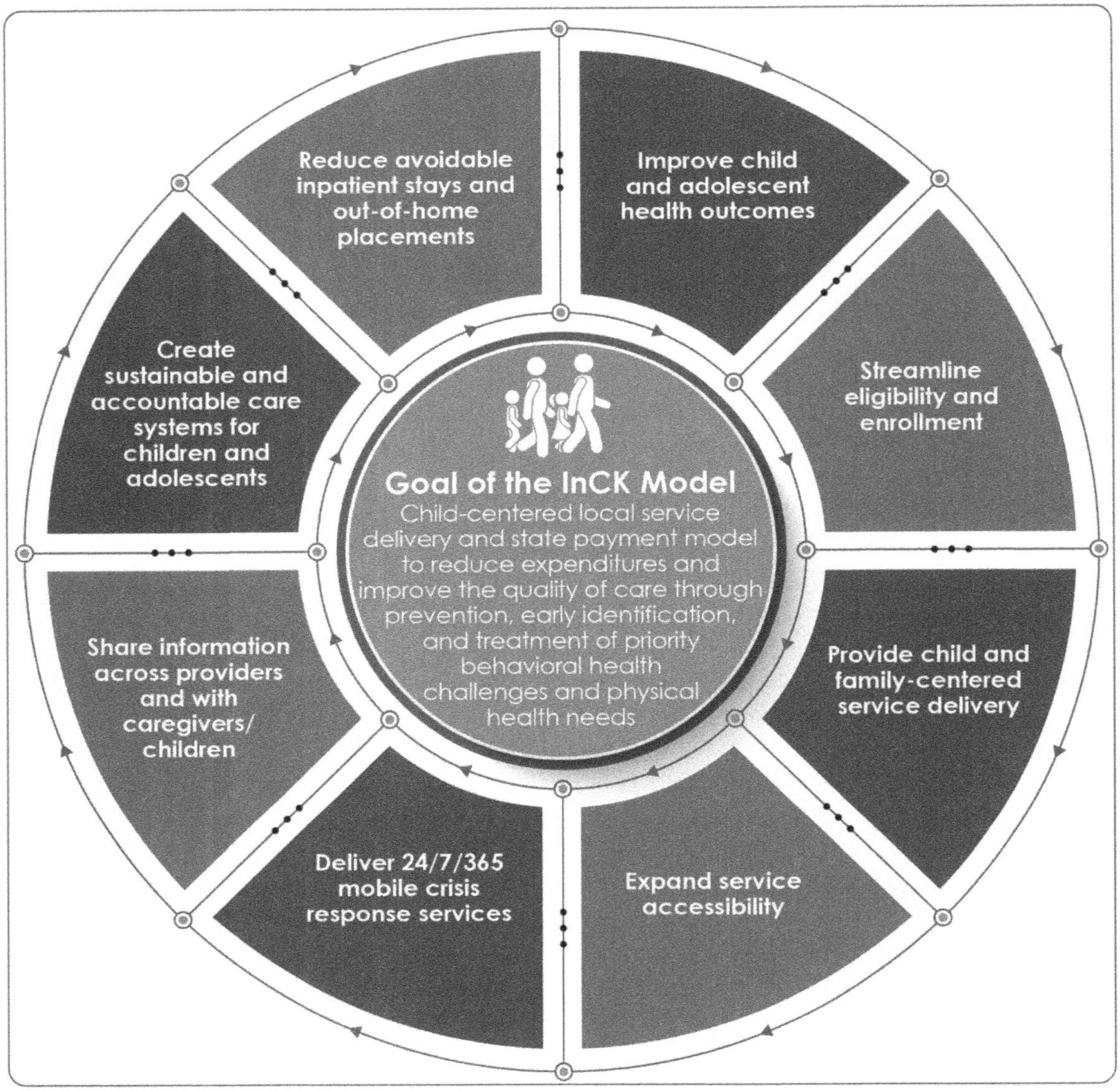

Figure 3-1. The Integrated Care for Kids Model

Reproduced from Abt Associates Inc. *Integrated Care for Kids (InCK) Model Evaluation: Report 1*. August 23, 2022. Accessed June 3, 2024. https://www.cms.gov/priorities/innovation/data-and-reports/2022/inck-model-pre-imp-first-eval-rpt.

North Carolina InCK (NC InCK) launched for all Medicaid-insured children, adolescents, and adults from birth to 20 years of age in 5 counties in January 2022. Beneficiaries who face increased risk will have access to additional support through their Family Navigator and cross-sector care team members, who will create shared action plans with families. The NC InCK APM promotes child-centered care by linking payment to the delivery of high-quality care, such as assessing kindergarten readiness and screening for food insecurity. For example, practices receive financial incentives for discussing community literacy resources or prekindergarten options with parents.

Key Concept

Alternative payment models involve direct funding of interventions that address HRSNs. Among them, ACOs and AHCs are 2 such initiatives that have found success with primarily adult populations. The InCK Model is a child-centered APM focused on the early identification and treatment of behavioral and social needs of children.

Screening in Different Settings

The nonclinical factors that contribute to an individual's well-being are extensive and often overlap, including housing and/or food insecurity, lack of transportation, and inability to afford medications. Medical organizations that previously outlined purely clinical guidelines to help determine diagnosis and management of health conditions have come to accept and promote HRSNs as important factors in patient health. The federal and state governments have created and implemented pathways for financing and reimbursement of initiatives focused on ameliorating HRSNs. Subsequently, this support has incentivized health systems and health care professionals to incorporate screening for HRSNs and creation of road maps to address HRSNs as part of routine patient care. Regarding screening, numerous research studies have examined ideal screening practices in various settings, such as outpatient primary care and subspecialty clinics, EDs, and inpatient units, including frequency of screening and populations to screen. Frequency of screening can vary from once at initial contact, to annually, to perhaps even at every point of contact with the patient. Health care professionals may choose to screen only the populations at highest risk (eg, patients with>2 visits to the ED annually) or to screen only children of certain ages, such as newborns, depending on capacity. Screening can take place via self-administered paper forms or tablet-based questionnaires or, alternatively, be administered by the provider in the examination room as part of the visit. These decisions need to take into consideration varying levels of support staff and resources as well as barriers to screening that may exist within a particular setting or for a particular population.

At the practice level, meeting the identified needs of the patient or family can take on various forms. Resource lists (compiled by a volunteer or by the health care staff) are low in cost, although they may require constant upkeep. With use of the EHR in most health care settings, these lists can be incorporated into the EHR and easily shared with families. Many states and cities have compiled free online directories searchable by zip code, which are periodically updated. In-person assistance at the time a need is identified is ideal. Social workers have an educational background in social care, while community health workers can act as a cultural bridge between a health care setting and a community. Case managers, care managers, and psychologists can also meet the HRSNs of patients, especially those with complex medical or behavioral conditions. Programs such as Health Leads use college-aged volunteers to contact patients who need assistance connecting to community resources. Although Health Leads may be unavailable in your area, there is always the option of using undergraduate students, who are interested in health care, as volunteers.

Summary

Health-related social needs are now widely recognized by professional health care organizations as essential for ensuring positive health outcomes for patients, regardless of the medical field. Governmental agencies at all levels have financing mechanisms available to support the incorporation of HRSNs into clinical care. It is within the capacity of health care systems, hospitals, and outpatient practices not only to screen for HRSNs but to establish processes by which these needs can be addressed once identified, to positively influence the health and well-being of communities and patients.

Key Points

- The recognition that HRSNs influence downstream health outcomes is transforming clinical practice across all settings.
- Various professional health care organizations have put forth policy statements on the importance of recognizing and addressing HRSNs to positively influence health.
- Professional organization guidelines include discussion of social needs as well as recommendations for how lawmakers and health systems should address these social needs.
- In growing recognition of HRSNs, federal and state agencies have proposed various means of financing mechanisms to incentivize and reimburse state-level initiatives and programming.

References

1. Brooks-Gunn J, Duncan GJ. The effects of poverty on children. *Future Child*. 1997;7(2):55–71 PMID: 9299837 doi: 10.2307/1602387
2. Boyle CA, Boulet S, Schieve LA, et al. Trends in the prevalence of developmental disabilities in US children, 1997–2008. *Pediatrics*. 2011;127(6):1034–1042 PMID: 21606152 doi: 10.1542/peds.2010-2989
3. Blair C, Granger DA, Willoughby M, et al; FLP Investigators. Salivary cortisol mediates effects of poverty and parenting on executive functions in early childhood. *Child Dev*. 2011;82(6):1970–1984 PMID: 22026915 doi: 10.1111/j.1467-8624.2011.01643.x
4. Shonkoff JP, Garner AS, Siegel BS, et al; American Academy of Pediatrics Committee on Psychosocial Aspects of Child and Family Health; Committee on Early Childhood, Adoption, and Dependent Care; and Section on Developmental and Behavioral Pediatrics. The lifelong effects of early childhood adversity and toxic stress. *Pediatrics*. 2012;129(1):e232–e246 PMID: 22201156 doi: 10.1542/peds.2011-2663
5. Belfield CR, Levin HM, eds. *The Price We Pay: Economic and Social Consequences of Inadequate Education*. Brookings Press; 2007
6. Isaacs JB. International comparisons of economic mobility. In: Isaacs JB, Sawhill IV, Haskins R, eds. *Getting Ahead or Losing Ground: Economic Mobility in America*. Brookings Institution; 2008:37–44
7. Gitterman BA, Flanagan PJ, Cotton WH, et al; American Academy of Pediatrics Council on Community Pediatrics. Poverty and child health in the United States. *Pediatrics*. 2016;137(4):e20160339 PMID: 26962238 doi: 10.1542/peds.2016-0339
8. American Academy of Pediatrics. Bright Futures. Accessed April 15, 2024. https://www.aap.org/en/practice-management/bright-futures
9. Chung EK, Siegel BS, Garg A, et al. Screening for social determinants of health among children and families living in poverty: a guide for clinicians. *Curr Probl Pediatr Adolesc Health Care*. 2016;46(5):135–153 PMID: 27101890 doi: 10.1016/j.cppeds.2016.02.004

10. Daniel H, Bornstein SS, Kane GC; Health and Public Policy Committee of the American College of Physicians. Addressing social determinants to improve patient care and promote health equity: an American College of Physicians position paper. *Ann Intern Med.* 2018;168(8):577–578 PMID: 29677265 doi: 10.7326/M17-2441
11. Ades V, Goddard B, Pearson Ayala S, Chemouni Bach S, Wu SX. ACOG committee opinion No. 729: importance of social determinants of health and cultural awareness in the delivery of reproductive health care. *Obstet Gynecol.* 2018;131(6):1162–1163 PMID: 29794658 doi: 10.1097/AOG.0000000000002660
12. American Academy of Family Physicians. Advancing health equity by addressing the social determinants of health in family medicine (position paper). Accessed April 16, 2024. https://www.aafp.org/about/policies/all/social-determinants-health-family-medicine-position-paper.html
13. National Academies of Science, Engineering, and Medicine. Integrating social care into the delivery of health care: moving upstream to improve the nation's health. 2019. Accessed April 16, 2024. https://nap.nationalacademies.org/catalog/25467/integrating-social-care-into-the-delivery-of-health-care-moving
14. Centers for Medicare & Medicaid Services. Early and Periodic Screening, Diagnostic, and Treatment. Medicaid.gov. Accessed April 17, 2024. https://www.medicaid.gov/medicaid/benefits/early-and-periodic-screening-diagnostic-and-treatment/index.html
15. Tsai D. RE: additional guidance on use of in lieu of services and settings in Medicaid managed care. US Department of Health and Human Services. January 4, 2023. Accessed April 17, 2024. https://www.medicaid.gov/sites/default/files/2023-01/smd23001.pdf
16. *Medi-Cal Community Supports, or In Lieu of Services (ILOS), Policy Guide.* California Dept of Health Care Services; 2023. Accessed April 17, 2024. https://www.dhcs.ca.gov/Documents/MCQMD/DHCS-Community-Supports-Policy-Guide.pdf
17. Kaiser Family Foundation. Medicaid waiver tracker: approved and pending Section 1115 waivers by state. Accessed September 11, 2024. https://www.kff.org/medicaid/issue-brief/medicaid-waiver-tracker-approved-and-pending-section-1115-waivers-by-state
18. Centers for Medicare & Medicaid Services. North Carolina Medicaid Reform Demonstration. Medicaid.gov. Accessed April 17, 2024. https://www.medicaid.gov/medicaid/section-1115-demo/demonstration-and-waiver-list/82766
19. Centers for Medicare & Medicaid Services. California Advancing and Innovating Medi-Cal (CalAIM). Medicaid.gov. Accessed April 17, 2024. https://www.medicaid.gov/medicaid/section-1115-demo/demonstration-and-waiver-list/81046
20. National Association of ACOs. Medicaid ACOs. Accessed October 1, 2024. https://www.naacos.com/medicaid
21. CMS.gov. Accountable Health Communities Model. Accessed April 17, 2024. https://innovation.cms.gov/innovation-models/ahcm
22. Johnson KA, Barolin N, Ogbue C, Verlander K. Lessons from five years of the CMS Accountable Health Communities Model. *Health Affairs Forefront* blog. August 8, 2022. Accessed April 17, 2024. https://www.healthaffairs.org/content/forefront/lessons-five-years-cms-accountable-health-communities-model
23. CMS.gov. Integrated Care for Kids (InCK) Model. Accessed April 17, 2024. https://innovation.cms.gov/innovation-models/integrated-care-for-kids-model

CHAPTER 4

Screening for Social Needs in the Pediatric Clinical Setting

Hemen Muleta, MD, FAAP; Dana Sanderson, MD; and Jenna Scholnick, MD, FAAP

Screening for the social determinants of health (SDOH) is recognized as an important practice that pediatric health care professionals are expected to perform. Although there is agreement about the importance of the practice, there is no standard for implementing social needs screening in the clinical setting. Important considerations in developing a screening program include selecting a social needs screening tool, enlisting trained staff, and creating a workflow for collecting, documenting, and responding to patients' social needs. Developing a resource referral system for families that disclose social needs is particularly important to build a trusting relationship with families, normalize screening across a health system, and, through intervention, reduce these needs. As the field grows, several regulatory, billing, and funding changes are also emerging in support of expanding SDOH screening and responses.

CHAPTER 4

Screening for Social Needs in the Pediatric Clinical Setting

Hemen Muleta, MD, FAAP; Dana Sanderson, MD; and Jenna Scholnick, MD, FAAP

Introduction/Why Screening for Social Needs Is Important

It is well recognized that social determinants of health (SDOH; also referred to as *social drivers of health*) and health-related social needs (HRSNs) have significant roles in a person's health outcomes. Without a systematic process for screening within the clinical setting, however, patients' needs may go unidentified.

In 2016, the American Academy of Pediatrics (AAP) released a policy statement making a strong recommendation for SDOH screening in pediatric health care settings and appropriate linkage to community resources.[1] This recommendation emerged from the understanding that detecting social needs and providing means to ameliorate the impact on families will lead to improved health outcomes. Since the release of this initial AAP policy statement, numerous other professional organizations have also endorsed the need for SDOH screening in clinical settings. These organizations include the American College of Obstetricians and Gynecologists,[2] American Academy of Family Physicians,[3] Academic Pediatric Association,[4] National Academy of Medicine,[5] American College of Physicians,[6] and National Academies of Science, Engineering, and Medicine.[7] Their work is detailed in the Professional Health Care Organization Policy Statements section of Chapter 3, Guidelines and Policies for Integrating Social Care Into Clinical Practice.

Although it is challenging to estimate the prevalence of SDOH screening in health care systems across the United States, research efforts and publications around SDOH screening have grown exponentially over the past decade. These studies have reported on critical findings, including the perspectives of community members and program participants, the modalities of screening currently available, and the barriers and facilitators of SDOH screening in various clinical settings. Overall, these studies have shown that health care professionals find SDOH screening important, and screening is welcomed by families.[8–10] Furthermore, caregivers of pediatric patients screened for unmet social needs by pediatric professionals form favorable views of the health care team.[9] Data thus far from various studies focused on SDOH screening have shown promising outcomes. Social determinants of health screening can elucidate the level and type of needs that exist within a community. Screening and intervention programs can lead to increased referrals to community resources and improvements in social needs.[11] Such interventions can also positively influence health outcomes, such as enhancing vaccination participation, decreasing hospitalization rates, reducing asthma risk factors, and improving caregiver-reported health status.[12,13]

While the initial focus of social needs screening has been on outpatient settings, there is increasing understanding among health care professionals that SDOH screening is also important in patients who have been hospitalized. The hospitalization of a child can be an acute and unexpected stressor for families, putting them at a higher risk for HRSNs caused by missed wages and hospital bills. In one study of hospitalized children, 25% of the surveyed families were food insecure and a large percentage were not connected to resources they likely qualified for, such as the Supplemental Nutrition Assistance Program (SNAP) and the Supplemental Nutrition Program for Women, Infants, and Children (WIC).[14] The inpatient setting can also be a venue for supporting patients with social needs who are not linked with ambulatory clinics, have been lost to follow-up, or do not have access to outpatient care.

The next section discusses the currently available SDOH screening tools and how to select a screening tool based on the health care context and patient needs.

Key Concept

Research studies on social needs assessment and interventions have shown the ability of health care professionals to understand the needs of their patients, link patients to community resources, and positively influence health outcomes.

Overview of Available Social Determinants of Health Screening Tools

To determine which screening tool to use, clinicians should understand the domains of SDOH. The Centers for Medicare & Medicaid Services (CMS) outlines 5 domains[15]:

- Food insecurity
- Housing instability
- Utility needs
- Transportation needs
- Interpersonal violence

Additional areas to consider, which have been highlighted by the most recent update from the CMS and by the broad HRSN literature, include job access, financial constraints, legal needs, immigration status, child care, social support, stress, substance use treatment, and educational opportunities. Social needs screening using a standardized questionnaire is one tool the pediatrician can use to detect potential social issues. Another proposed mechanism has been to incorporate SDOH questions throughout the social history of a patient encounter.

In general, the selection of the screening tool should be tailored to the needs of the community, the availability and training of staff, and the capacity and resources of the clinical setting, institution, and community.[16] Generalized screening tools can be chosen that detect multiple social needs, or more tailored screening tools can be chosen that detect specific domains. Ideally, the screening tool should be validated and evidence based. Given the relative novelty of the field, however, psychometric and pragmatic validity of the screening tools is often tested as part of the implementation process by health care systems. Screening tools should be easy to understand and available in multiple languages to meet the needs of the patient population. The overall length and duration of the questionnaire, and the modes of administration that it is validated for, should also be considered.

Key Concept

Important considerations to keep in mind when selecting a social needs screening tool include the scope of social need domains assessed by the screening tool, based on community needs and available resources; the reliability and validity within the target population; availability at an appropriate reading level and translations into languages specific to the community; and the length, durations, and modes of administration of the screening tool.

Multiple screening tools are now available for the pediatric and general patient populations. **Table 4-1** summarizes and compares the most commonly encountered screening tools, adapted from the Social Interventions Research & Evaluation Network (SIREN).[17] A more detailed and routinely updated screening tools comparison table can be found on the SIREN Evidence & Resource Library website (https://sirenetwork.ucsf.edu/tools/evidence-library). In collaboration with Kaiser Permanente, SIREN also hosts an interactive website through which health care professionals can search for screening tools based on social need domains of interest.[18] **Figures 4-1** and **4-2** provide examples of commonly used screening tools.

Developing a Social Needs Screening Program

Although there is agreement among pediatricians and health care quality leaders about the importance of screening for social needs, there is no standardized workflow across pediatric settings. However, several guidelines and best practices have been published to assist clinicians and health care systems.[4,19] Each clinical practice should assess how to operationalize a social needs screening program. Next, we present a discussion about strategies and factors to consider when developing a screening program.

Approach to Implementation

There are benefits to developing a screening process through an implementation science or quality improvement (QI) lens. In the clinical setting, it allows for a means of evaluating the reach, acceptability, and sustainability of the program. It also allows for changes to be made within the screening process. A few important measures to consider include, but are not limited to, the percentage of families screened, the barriers and facilitators identified in the workflow, and the duration and time required of families and staff to complete the screening tool. Common models of implementation and evaluation include the Reach, Effectiveness, Adoption, Implementation, or Maintenance framework.[20] Another potential implementation and assessment approach that

Table 4-1. Summary of Commonly Available Social Determinants of Health Screening Tools[a]

Screening Tool	Population	Administration Methods	Duration, min	No. of SDOH Questions	Various Languages	SDOH Domains					
						Food Insecurity	Housing	Utilities	Transportation	Interpersonal Violence	Others
WE CARE[b]	Pediatric	Self	<5	6–15	✓	✓	✓	✓			Child care, education, employment
I-HELP[c]	Pediatric	Staff	30	14		✓	✓			✓	Education, financial constraints, health care access, immigration, legal needs
iScreen[d]	Pediatric	Self or staff	10	23	✓						
SEEK[e]	Pediatric	Self	3	9	✓	✓				✓	Social support, stress
SWYC[f]	Pediatric		10	9		✓				✓	
HelpSteps[g]	Pediatric/ young adult	Self	25	90–166		✓	✓			✓	Education, health care access, income, physical activity, substance use
AHC[h]	All ages	Self or staff	2	19		✓	✓	✓	✓	✓	Disabilities, education, employment, financial constraints, social support, stress
Health Leads[i]	All ages	Self	<5	10	✓	✓	✓	✓	✓		Child care, health care access, literacy, social support
HealthBegins[j]	All ages	Staff	6	24		✓	✓		✓	✓	Education, employment, financial constraints, neighborhood safety, immigration, social support, stress
PRAPARE[k]	All ages	Staff	11	17	✓	✓	✓	✓	✓	✓	Child care, clothing, education, employment, health care access, immigration, incarceration, income, neighborhood safety, social support, stress
WellRx[l]	All ages	Self or staff	NR	10	✓	✓	✓	✓	✓	✓	Child care, education, employment, neighborhood safety
AAFP[m]	All ages	Self or staff		15		✓	✓	✓	✓	✓	Child care, education, employment, financial constraints

YCLS[n]	All ages	Self or staff	NR	10		✓	✓	✓	✓	✓	Child care, financial constraints, health care access, literacy, neighborhood safety, social support, stress
Medicare Total Health Assessment[o]	All ages	Self or staff	10–20	9		✓	✓				Legal needs, social support, stress
THRIVE[p]	Adult	Self	NR	11		✓	✓	✓	✓		Education, employment, health care access,
NAM[q]	Adult	Self	5	12						✓	Education, financial constraints, income, social support, stress

Abbreviations: AAFP, American Academy of Family Physicians; AHC, Accountable Health Communities; I-HELP, income, housing and utilities, education and employment, legal status, and personal and family stability; NAM, National Academy of Medicine; NR, not reported; PRAPARE, Protocol for Responding to and Assessing Patients' Assets, Risks and Experience; SDOH, social determinants of health; SEEK, Safe Environment for Every Kid; SYWC, Survey of Well-being of Young Children; THRIVE, Tool for Health & Resilience in Vulnerable Environments; WE CARE, Well Child Care, Evaluation, Community Resources, Advocacy, Referral, Education; YCLS, Your Current Life Situation.

[a] Arranged by specificity of population, the screener tool was designed to assess from pediatrics, to all ages, to adults only.

[b] Garg A, Butz AM, Dworkin PH, Lewis RA, Thompson RE, Serwint JR. Improving the management of family psychosocial problems at low-income children's well-child care visits: the WE CARE Project. *Pediatrics*. 2007;120(3):547–558.

[c] Colvin JD, Bettenhausen JL, Anderson-Carpenter KD, Collie-Akers V, Chung PJ. Caregiver opinion of in-hospital screening for unmet social needs by pediatric residents. *Acad Pediatr*. 2016;16(2):161–167.

[d] Gottlieb L, Hessler D, Long D, Amaya A, Adler N. A randomized trial on screening for social determinants of health: the iScreen study. *Pediatrics*. 2014;134(6):e1611–e1618.

[e] Palinkas LA, Belanger R, Newton S, Saldana L, Landsverk J, Dubowitz H. Assessment of adoption and early implementation barriers and facilitators of the Safe Environment for Every Kid (SEEK) model. *Acad Pediatr*. 2023;23(7):1434–1445.

[f] Perrin EC, Sheldrick C, Visco Z, Mattern K. *The Survey of Well-being of Young Children (SWYC) User's Manual*. Floating Hospital for Children at Tufts Medical Center; 2016. Accessed April 24, 2024. https://www.tuftsmedicine.org/sites/default/files/2024-01/swyc-manual-v101-web-format-33016.pdf.

[g] Hassan A, Blood EA, Pikcilingis A, et al. Youths' health-related social problems: concerns often overlooked during the medical visit. *J Adolesc Health*. 2013;53(2):265–271.

[h] Beil H, Brower H, Chepaitis A, et al. *Accountable Health Communities (AHC) Model Evaluation: Second Evaluation Report*. Centers for Medicare & Medicaid; 2023. Accessed April 24, 2024. https://www.cms.gov/priorities/innovation/data-and-reports/2023/ahc-second-eval-rpt.

[i] The Health Leads Social Health Data Toolkit. Health Leads. Accessed April 25, 2024. https://healthleadsusa.org/news-resources/social-health-data-toolkit.

[j] Hensley C, Joseph A, Shah S, O'Dea C, Carameli K. Addressing social determinants of health at a federally qualified health center. *Int Public Health J*. 2017;9(2):189–198.

[k] The PRAPARE Screening Tool. PRAPARE. Accessed April 25, 2024. https://prapare.org/the-prapare-screening-tool.

[l] Page-Reeves J, Kaufman W, Bleecker M, et al. Addressing social determinants of health in a clinic setting: the WellRx pilot in Albuquerque, New Mexico. *J Am Board Fam Med*. 2016;29(3):414–418.

[m] The EveryONE Project. American Academy of Family Physicians. Accessed April 25, 2024. https://www.aafp.org/family-physician/patient-care/the-everyone-project.html.

[n] Kaiser Permanente. Your Current Life Situation (Shorter Form). Social Interventions Research & Evaluation Network. November 10, 2016. Accessed April 25, 2024. https://sirenetwork.ucsf.edu/sites/default/files/Your%20Current%20Life%20Situation%20Questionnaire%20v2-0%20%28Core%20and%20supplemental%29%20no%20highlights.pdf.

[o] Freedman D, VanderHorst N. Utilization of high-technology to collect health risk assessment information from Medicare members: a feasibility study of Interactive Voice Response (IVR) and an online survey tool. *Clin Med Res*. 2013;11(3):175–176.

[p] Buitron de la Vega P, Losi S, Sprague Martinez L, et al. Implementing an EHR-based screening and referral system to address social determinants of health in primary care. *Med Care*. 2019;57(6)(suppl 2):S133–S139.

[q] Giuse NB, Koonce TY, Kusnoor SV, et al. Institute of Medicine measures of social and behavioral determinants of health: a feasibility study. *Am J Prev Med*. 2017;52(2):199–206.

	Yes/No
In the last 12 months,[a] did you ever **eat less than you felt you should** because there wasn't enough money for food?	Y N
In the last 12 months, has the **electric, gas, oil, or water company threatened to shut off your services** in your home?	Y N
Are you worried that in the next 2 months, you **may not have stable housing?**	Y N
Do problems getting **child care make it difficult for you to work or study?** *(leave blank if you do not have children)*	Y N
In the last 12 months, have you needed to see a doctor, **but could not because of cost?**	Y N
In the last 12 months, have you ever had to go without health care because you didn't have **a way to get there?**	Y N
Do you ever need help **reading hospital materials?**	Y N
Do you often feel that **you lack companionship?**	Y N
Are any of your needs urgent? For example: I don't have food tonight, I don't have a place to sleep tonight	Y N
If you checked YES to any boxes above, **would you like to receive assistance** with any of these needs?	Y N

Figure 4-1. The Health Leads Screening Tool

[a] Time frames can be altered as needed.

From The Health Leads Social Health Data Toolkit. Health Leads. Accessed April 25, 2024. https://healthleadsusa.org/news-resources/social-health-data-toolkit.

can be used is the Practical Robust Implementation and Sustainability Model.[21] Additionally, the implementation could be approached through the QI lens of Plan-Do-Study-Act cycles.[22]

Regardless of the method of choice, such a systematic approach allows for ongoing improvements in the screening process, reiteration and expansion of the program to other clinical settings, and dissemination of findings to help inform best practices to assist clinicians and health care systems at large.

Training Health Care Staff Members

Once the implementation plan is established, all staff members should be trained in the importance of SDOH, the screening process, and the delivery of trauma-informed care. They should also be trained in recognizing their potential for bias when interacting with families with documented social needs. The screening and intervention process should be conducted in an empathetic and sensitive manner with attention to the privacy of the family. The RESPECT (respect, explanatory model, social context, power, empathy, concerns, and trust/team) model is a widely used framework for improving communication during patient care.[23] The premise of this model

Do you have a high school degree?	Yes No ↓ If NO, would you like help to get a GED?	Yes No Maybe Later
Do you have a job?	Yes No ↓ If NO, would you like help with finding employment and/or job training?	Yes No Maybe Later
Do you need daycare for your child?	Yes No ↓ If YES, would you like help finding it?	Yes No Maybe Later
Do you think you are at risk of becoming homeless?	Yes No ↓ If YES, would you like help with this?	Yes No Maybe Later ↓ If yes, is this an emergency? Yes* No
Do you always have enough food for your family?	Yes No ↓ If NO, would you like help with this?	Yes No Maybe Later ↓ If yes, do you need food for tonight? Yes* No
Do you have trouble paying your heating bill and/or electricity bill?	Yes No ↓ If YES, would you like help with this?	Yes No Maybe Later ↓ If yes, are you at risk of having your utilities shut off in the next week? Yes* No

Parent Name: ______________________ **Phone:** ______________ *Patient is eligible for immediate referral to Health Leads

Figure 4-2. The WE CARE Screening Tool

WE CARE indicates Well Child Care, Evaluation, Community Resources, Advocacy, Referral, Education. Reproduced with permission from Arvin Garg, MD, MPH, FAAP.

is to establish rapport with patients, empathize with them, and support and partner with them based on where they are in their desire or readiness to accept assistance. This will help with patient comfortableness and openness in disclosing needs, which will further the clinician's ability to assist with those needs.[24]

Establishing a safe and private environment can improve patients' trust in the health care professional. It is best to introduce the screening questionnaire with assurances that the questions are asked of everyone and that the answers are kept confidential. This way, the screening is normalized as a standard of care for all patients and families. A simple explanation of the connection between one's medical health and emotional health may also be helpful to patients. This can be a written statement before the first question on the screening tool or a verbal statement from the person doing the screening. Frequent eye contact and facing the patient while leaning in slightly, with occasional nods, are ways to convey interest and engagement. Using interpreters to overcome language barriers is essential to providing culturally effective care.

It is important to express appreciation if a patient discloses a difficult experience and to provide empathetic statements that acknowledge hardships they have faced. A motivational interviewing approach can be used to ask about the family's priority for social needs assistance, allowing them to express which needs they find most pressing and helping them set tangible goals. Additionally, health care professionals should use a strengths-based approach when discussing social needs with families. Identifying protective family and social supports is essential, as these are often used to buffer adverse social factors, especially those related to children and their health, and can help promote positive attitudes and behaviors in caregivers.[23]

Developing a Workflow

Part of the staff training should include a thorough understanding of the HRSN screening and response process. Collaborators from various departments must have input in the screening workflow. Clinicians, nurses, front desk staff, community health workers (CHWs), parents, and administrative staff should collaborate to create a workflow. The workflow should outline the appropriate roles of all team members and should ideally be integrated into the existing structure of the health care setting. Process mapping can help visualize the workflow as it is and how it should be and steps to improve on. For screening to flow smoothly, the process should be streamlined, wasteful activities should be eliminated, and staff and health care professionals should work efficiently and at their highest level of training. It is also helpful to consider how other successful screening programs were implemented and are functioning. If there are other screening activities already being conducted in the clinical setting, it might make sense to include the SDOH screening within the already established workflow. For example, for primary care offices, the screening tool could be part of a larger packet of surveys, such as the Modified Checklist for Autism in Toddlers or the Ages & Stages Questionnaires, that families and staff are already familiar with. Establishing in advance which staff members have the role of providing/administering the screening tool, documenting results, discussing results with families, and providing the necessary interventions can also help the SDOH screening become a routine aspect of the clinical practice. Regular team meetings should be set up to discuss, review, and modify the workflow.

In the hospital setting, the workflow should be tailored to the circumstances and special challenges these settings present. For example, in the emergency department (ED), screening could be incorporated into the registration process when demographic data are provided at patient presentation. For inpatient care, the screening could be part of the admission process in each unit. Screening could also be incorporated as part of a daily rounding checklist of items to be completed by the inpatient teams. The workflow may need to be altered to accommodate for the staffing composition and unique necessities of each hospital unit. Training should especially focus on ensuring that evening and weekend staff members as well as rotating staff, such as residents, are also well-versed in the workflow. Interdisciplinary or case management rounds, which tend to be a common part of the daily workflow in hospital units, can be used as an opportunity to review results if SDOH screenings have been completed, to identify patients for whom the screening tool still needs to be administered, and to recognize and provide resources for families that screen positive for needs.

Universal Screening

Implementing a screening program in clinical practice and establishing a workflow should ideally lead to the universal screening of all patients, which is important for many reasons. Most social needs are not evident when meeting a patient and their family. Standardized screening is an excellent supplement to the social history that is usually collected during patient interaction and often includes more open-ended questions. Furthermore, if all patients are screened according to a universal protocol, there is less concern for stigmatizing individuals when asking about potentially sensitive topics.[4] As important as universal screening is, providing families the option to opt out of screening is also necessary to respect the privacy and autonomy of patients and families.

Targeted screening at annual health supervision visits, at new patient visits, at certain ages, or while caring for patients with chronic diseases (eg, asthma) can help establish a screening routine and prevent screening fatigue. Screening should be performed at regular intervals, as the social needs of families with socioeconomic challenges are often changing.[19]

Repeated screening is especially important for patients with certain chronic diseases, such as asthma. In fact, screening and addressing social needs has been shown to reduce ED visits and admissions for asthma, one of the most common causes of hospitalization in children.[25] The acuity of an ED visit and subsequent admission can also lead to an exacerbation of certain social needs and therefore necessitates SDOH screening at each isolated ED encounter or admission. Exceptions should of course be made based on unique circumstances to reduce screening fatigue by families.

Modality of Screening

To an extent, this depends on the type of screening tool being used. For example, the Health Leads questionnaire is validated for self-administration, while the I-HELP questions are specifically designed for a health care professional to incorporate into the social history of a patient encounter.[9,26] Regarding patient privacy, there is some evidence to indicate that patients are more likely to disclose needs through an electronic-based, self-administered questionnaire than face-to-face verbal screening.[27] Studies that have specifically looked at patient preferences have reported mixed results; some studies have shown a preference for being screened privately, while others have reported comfortableness in being screened by health care professionals.[28,29] The current evidence does not seem to show a strong preference from families on which staff member (nurse, doctor, or social worker) should conduct the screening.[28]

The balance between privacy and administration is also relevant when deciding between electronic and paper screening. One advantage of an electronic-based screening tool is the ability for families to complete the questionnaire privately, which, as previously mentioned, may improve self-disclosure. This is especially advantageous if the screening questions are integrated with the patient's electronic health record (EHR), allowing health care professionals to review and document the results over time. Patients could complete their questionnaire via their patient portal before the visit. Clinical staff can work with families that have limited access to the internet or that need literacy/language assistance to complete the questionnaire. The option for parents to access their child's EHR may be restricted as a result of confidentiality policies related to adolescent patients.

Another electronic option is to have screening questions available on tablets during a clinical encounter or hospital admission, with clinical staff on hand to assist families that have challenges related to language barriers, literacy, and disability. Paper-based screening questionnaires remain common given their ease of accessibility and low resource need. However, paper screeners may be easily misplaced, require staff time to administer and transcribe to the EHR, and may be incorrectly transcribed to the EHR. Overall, to achieve the goal of universal screening, clinical settings may need to combine various modalities of screening. This may mean allowing those who can access their patient portals to complete the screening through their EHR, providing a tablet- or paper-based screening tool for those who do not have a patient portal, and, finally, having clinic staff verbally assist patients who cannot complete the questions independently for the variety of reasons previously discussed.

Key Concept

The modality used for social needs screening partially depends on the health care setting and the capabilities of its EHR. Several screening modalities may need to be implemented to take into account patients with various technological access, language needs and reading levels, and accessibility needs.

Documenting Screening Results

Unique challenges arise with the increase in social needs screening in organizations across the country alongside efforts to increase transparency of patient information through the 21st Century Cures Act. Through the act, health care organizations are now mandated to electronically release clinical documents to patients as soon as they are finalized.[30] Health care systems need to ensure that social needs data are obtained, documented, and shared thoughtfully, as this important information becomes part of the patient health record.[19] Incorrect handling of this sensitive information may affect patient-provider trust, violate patient confidentiality, and lead to bias during clinical care. There is no standard for how and where screening data are collected. As discussed in the Modality of Screening section earlier in this chapter, organizations may collect patient data electronically, on paper, or verbally.

Institutional policies for documenting social needs data in the EHR should be transparent. One recent study of parents of hospitalized children who screened positive for HRSNs showed that families accepted documentation of this information in the EHR if used to provide them with resources and if done in a transparent manner.[31] Families should be given the option to opt out of having their social needs results documented in the health record. Some families may feel comfortable with their child's pediatrician knowing this information but object to other health care professionals knowing or to the results being included in the EHR. Thought also needs to be given to sensitive information that one caregiver may not want shared with another caregiver, including how this can be documented in a secure fashion to prevent unwanted disclosure of information.[24]

Large hospital systems with well-staffed information technology teams may find it easier than small clinics to integrate screening data into the EHR. Consideration needs to be given to where in the EHR the data will go so the workflow can be streamlined for health care professionals. The data should be easily visible and accessible for the clinician to act on the results. In an inpatient setting, it might make the most sense for a template note to be provided so SDOH results can be documented in a consistent manner, as several notes about the patient (eg, history and physical examination findings, progress note, discharge summary) will be documented during the admission. Data collected in the EHR can be used at an individual patient level, as well as at a population level, to quantify social and health disparities, to study implementation efforts, and to track results.[19]

Responding to Screening Results

It is important to have a response plan for families that screen positive for social needs. Screening results should trigger a conversation about a family's experiences, the family's current needs, and its priorities. Patients should never be automatically referred to a social care worker or program after a positive screening result. Rather, families should be asked whether they would like assistance for their unmet needs. For families that have social needs and are interested in receiving assistance, connecting them to appropriate resources is a crucial component of a successful screening and referrals program. Furthermore, it should be ensured that if a family is being referred to a community organization, there is sufficient capacity for the organization to respond to the patient's needs.[32] Failure to do so can decrease trust in the health care professionals and organization.

The response to a positive screening result depends on the capacity of the clinical setting and can include provision of resource sheets, referrals to staff with expertise in social needs, or adaptation of a colocation model with community organizations. As a first step, families can be provided with a routinely updated resource packet, which provides a list of community organizations and programs specific to the unmet social needs. Numerous online platforms also exist, including FindHelp and HITE, that can assist health care professionals in searching for electronic referrals based on location and domains of social needs.[33,34] Many of these platforms allow bidirectional communication between the person referring and the community organization receiving the referral. In some cases, it may even be possible to have these online platforms directly linked within an EHR system.

Another common response model is to refer patients with positive screening results to social workers, CHWs, or patient navigators who will then assist families in finding available resources. For example, the social care workforce may refer families to community-based resources such as food pantries, SNAP/WIC intake centers, child care providers, and employment, housing, or legal service organizations. Community health workers have specific training on addressing social needs and can follow up with patients over the course of weeks to months to ensure the family is equipped with all the information they need to participate in the assistance program. Studies have shown that deploying CHWs can increase the ability of families to be connected to resources in the outpatient and inpatient health care settings.[35,36] Additionally, such a navigation model has shown the potential to improve the caregiver-reported overall health of children.[12] This topic is covered more in the In-Person Support section of Chapter 8, Social Care Interventions.

Some health systems may also choose to develop a colocation of services model. In this model, the medical home would house additional services, such as a food pantry, a WIC enrollment office, or legal services. Medical-legal partnerships that advocate for patients by involving the legal system to improve housing, utility, immigration status, and public benefits have positively influenced outcomes.[37] This topic is covered more in the Partnerships section of Chapter 8.

Key Concept

Before the initiation of a social needs screening process, important considerations should be given to how positive social needs should be addressed. Collaborating with social care workforce and community-based organizations and integrating resource referral systems within an EHR are some examples of how to respond to social needs.

Barriers to Screening

While most health care professionals agree that screening for SDOH is important, a recent study showed that less than half of clinicians expressed confidence in their ability to address social needs and less than a quarter routinely screened for social needs.[8] Barriers to screening include lack of time, lack of training, and lack of comfort by health care professionals and staff. Furthermore, health care professionals are also at times unable to provide assistance as a result of limitations in community resources to address long-standing, complex social conditions.[21]

Patient discomfort, including a lack of trust in the health care professional and/or health care system, is an additional barrier to screening. Families fear facing stigma and bias from health care professionals. Families also cite that disclosing a need without being provided resources can be an added frustration.[10] The importance of building trust with patients on both individual and institutional levels cannot be overstated. Normalizing screening, clarifying the connection between social needs and health care, and effectively addressing patients' social needs can lessen these barriers.[19]

Health systems also need to be equipped to address urgent matters disclosed through SDOH screening, such as interpersonal violence, which may require acute intervention and escalation of reporting. The screening workflow should therefore include a mechanism for timely and appropriate responses to acute safety concerns. In accordance with the 21st Century Cures Act, careful consideration should also be given to what documentation is accessible to caregivers that may inadvertently affect patients and families.

The inpatient perspective also creates a few unique barriers to screening. These include times of staff shortages, high census, or high acuity that may deter staff from fully engaging in the screening workflow. Screening may also be deprioritized during nights and weekends when staffing in the hospital is decreased and referral services may not be available. Families may also not be ready to discuss social needs at a time of heightened stress and emotional vulnerability while caring for a sick child. This may be especially true in intensive care units (ICU), although further research is needed in ICU settings to determine so.

Key Concept

Commonly encountered barriers to implementing a social needs screening include unfamiliarity with how to screen, lack of time, worry over offending families through social questions, and concerns over limitations in available resources for positive screening results.

Evolution of the Social Determinants of Health Screening Landscape

As discussed in the introduction earlier in this chapter, SDOH screening and intervention has gained significant policy, clinical, and research interest.[20] Next, we highlight some exciting changes and progress that will improve the way SDOH screening is conducted across health care systems, payers, and professionals.

Regulatory Changes

In 2023, SDOH screening became a quality metric for the National Committee for Quality Assurance (NCQA) Healthcare Effectiveness Data and Information Set (HEDIS) for all patients.[38] HEDIS is used by most US health plans to measure patient care outcomes and quality of care. Specifically, the HEDIS metric measures focus on screening for food, housing, and transportation needs and on the response toward unmet social needs. Additionally, the NCQA highlights the expectation that health plans need to provide interventions to assist patients with positive SDOH screening results. Beginning in January 2024, the NCQA also requires health plans to provide performance reports on the SDOH quality metrics.[39] This incentivizes health plans to measure and work toward addressing health disparities within their patient populations.

In January 2023, The Joint Commission introduced new accreditation requirements for health care systems to identify HRSNs in adult patients and work to reduce racial and ethnic disparities in health outcomes. These requirements apply to hospitals, ambulatory primary care clinics, behavioral health centers, and human service organizations across all patient ages.[40] There are now requirements to assign a leader at each organization who oversees initiatives to address racial gaps in medical care, assess patients' HRSNs, and provide referrals and community resource information. Each organization has the flexibility to decide which patient populations and social domains to screen. Organizations are expected, however, to provide resources for patients with positive screening results.[39] Recognizing and addressing health care disparities is a marker of high-quality care that organizations are now expected to achieve to meet federal standards of care.

The CMS in 2022 released the updated *CMS Framework for Health Equity,* which details priorities to guide efforts in reducing health inequities and improving patient care within its programs.[41] Included in the priorities is the increased collection of patient-level demographic and SDOH data to understand patients' current needs within the 5 prioritized social need domains of food, housing, utilities, transportation, and interpersonal violence. This will inform priorities to further understand how current practices and policies contribute to health inequities, how to improve health care operations, and how to support the care of historically disinvested populations while working to reduce structural barriers to health. Beginning in January 2024, the CMS requires SDOH screening reports for hospitalized adults, ambulatory centers within the Medicare Merit-based Incentive Payment System, and all patients enrolled within Medicare Advantage Special Needs Plans.[39] A summary of the current regulatory standards can be found in **Table 4-2**.

Although these mandates are currently focused on an adult patient population, future iterations of the CMS requirements are likely to expand to children given that household-level social needs also influence pediatric health outcomes.

Billing Codes for Social Determinants of Health

Since 2015, *International Classification of Diseases, 10th Revision* (*ICD-10*), codes have expanded to include HRSN-specific Z codes (Z55–Z65), but these Z codes are still underutilized in US hospitals. Between 2016 and 2019, the utilization of HRSN-specific Z codes for hospitalized pediatric patients only slightly increased, from 1.4% to 1.9%.[42] Barriers likely contributing to this underutilization include lack of general knowledge of the availability of Z codes and their documentation requirements among health care professionals and health care coders. In most EHRs, the *ICD-10* Z codes also do not auto-populate when HRSN screening results are entered, further limiting their use. Until recently, SDOH results were not factored into the reimbursement model of billing, also contributing to their limited use. However, with the recent changes to the *Current Procedural Terminology* coding guidelines, if there is appropriate justification and explicit

Table 4-2. Current Social Needs Screening Regulatory Practices and Standards

Agency/ Organization (Program)	Social Care Quality Measures			Social Care–Related Regulations and Standards	
	NCQA (Healthcare Effectiveness Data and Information Set)	CMS (Hospital Inpatient Quality Reporting)	CMS (Merit-based Incentive Payment System)	CMS (Medicare Advantage Special Needs Plans' Health Risk Assessment)	The Joint Commission (Standard LD.04.03.08)
Description	Process measures: percentage of members screened at least once for 3 HRSNs and percentage of those who screened positive for 3 HRSNs and received a corresponding intervention, by domain	Health equity structural attestation measure: Does the hospital collect and document SDOH-related information from most of its patients, are needs documented in EHR structured fields, and are key performance indicators stratified by SDOH? Process measures: percentage of patients screened for 5 HRSNs and percentage of those who screened positive for 5 HRSNs	Process measure: percentage of patients screened for 5 HRSNs	Assessment must include ≥1 questions from the list of screening instruments on 3 HRSNs.	Organizations must screen hospitalized patients for HRSNs and provide information about community resources and support services.
Population	All ages	Adults aged ≥18 years	Adults aged ≥18 years	All plan enrollees	Representative sample or all patients
Setting	Health plans	Hospitals	Participating providers	Medicare Advantage Special Needs Plans	• All Critical Access Hospitals and hospitals • Ambulatory health care organizations • Behavioral health care and human service organizations
Domains	Food, housing, and transportation security	Food, housing, transportation, and utilities security; interpersonal violence	Food, housing, transportation, and utilities security; interpersonal violence	Food, housing, and transportation security	Organizations determine which HRSNs to include in assessment.
Intervention	Intervention on or up to 30 days after initial positive screening result	None required	None required	None specified	Required to provide information about community resources and support services
Instruments	Prespecified list of screening instruments	None specified	None specified	Prespecified list of screening instruments	None specified
Status	Process measure reporting only January 2023; performance reporting January 2024	Attestation reporting required January 2023; process measure reporting only January 2023; performance reporting January 2024	Voluntary reporting January 2023; performance reporting January 2024	Requirements begin in 2024.	Effective 2023

Abbreviations: CMS, Centers for Medicare & Medicaid Services; EHR, electronic health record; HRSN, health-related social need; NCQA, National Committee for Quality Assurance; SDOH, social determinants of health.

Adapted with permission from Gottlieb L, DeSilvey SC, Fichtenberg C, Bernheim S, Peltz A. Developing national social care standards. *Health Affairs Forefront* blog. February 22, 2023. Accessed April 25, 2024. https://www.healthaffairs.org/content/forefront/developing-national-social-care-standards.

documentation that a patient-reported HRSN significantly limits the diagnosis and treatment of the patient, HRSN-specific Z codes can be considered in the complexity of visits and medical decision-making in both ambulatory and inpatient settings.[43] As a next step, setting reimbursement standards for HRSN-specific Z codes will provide incentives for institutions to enhance their social needs screening program. Studies around documentation of Z codes and the effectiveness of the response of medical and social care teams are also needed.

Interventions to Address Positive Social Determinants of Health Screening Results

Over the past several years, both the CMS and private health plans have taken a robust interest and investment in interventions that address SDOH. For example, a study of private health insurances from 2017 to 2021 showed an increase in investment, especially for interventions that target housing and food insecurities.[44]

In 2017, the CMS created the Accountable Health Communities (AHC) Model through which participating clinical centers screen their patients and provide community resources to those deemed to have HRSNs or high utilization of ED services. In its latest report, the AHC Model shows promising results in reducing ED visits and community referrals, although it did not show a significant difference in actually obtaining resources.[15] Regardless, the AHC intervention provides a model for payers and health systems to follow. Future studies that focus on specific health outcomes and cost effectiveness will further elucidate the reach of the model.

The Section 1115 waivers are another example of a CMS program that address social needs. The Section 1115 waivers are typically used by states to implement new and innovative approaches to providing care for Medicaid beneficiaries, including nonmedical interventions for social needs. As of May 2024, 21 states have an 1115 waiver with HRSN provisions, with 16 states pending.[45]

As SDOH screening and interventions have recently garnered federal and national attention, the obligation of health care systems to screen and provide resources for their patients is also gaining wide acceptance as a standard of health care practice.

Key Points

- Social determinants of health screening is recommended across all pediatric health care settings, including outpatient clinics, EDs, and hospitals.
- Various screening tools are now available, and selection of an SDOH screening tool depends on the social need domains of interest and the capacity of each health system.
- A social needs screening and response program should be created with input and collaboration from key stakeholders. Such a program should ideally have measurable goals and be specific to the health system in place while providing a workflow that can be adapted for and expanded to additional clinical settings within the health system.
- Universal screening of patients using various modalities of screening is recommended to normalize screening and ensure that patients of different abilities can complete the screening.
- Developing a well–thought-out system to address social needs is necessary for an SDOH screening program to be effective and appropriately support patients.
- Several recent federal policy and regulatory changes have made SDOH screening a priority across health care systems and will likely lead to an acceleration in the study, reach, and outcomes of the field.

References

1. Gitterman BA, Flanagan PJ, Cotton WH, et al; American Academy of Pediatrics Council on Community Pediatrics. Poverty and child health in the United States. *Pediatrics.* 2016;137(4):e20160339 PMID: 26962238 doi: 10.1542/peds.2016-0339
2. Committee on Health Care for Underserved Women. ACOG committee opinion No. 729: importance of social determinants of health and cultural awareness in the delivery of reproductive health care. *Obstet Gynecol.* 2018;131(1):e43–e48 PMID: 29266079 doi:10.1097/AOG.0000000000002459
3. American Academy of Family Physicians. Advancing health equity by addressing the social determinants of health in family medicine (position paper). Accessed May 31, 2024. https://www.aafp.org/about/policies/all/social-determinants-health-family-medicine-position-paper.html
4. Chung EK, Siegel BS, Garg A, et al. Screening for social determinants of health among children and families living in poverty: a guide for clinicians. *Curr Probl Pediatr Adolesc Health Care.* 2016;46(5):135–153 PMID: 27101890 doi: 10.1016/j.cppeds.2016.02.004
5. Magnan S. Social determinants of health 201 for health care: plan, do, study, act. *NAM Perspect.* 2021;2021:10.31478/202106c PMID: 34532697 doi: 10.31478/202106c
6. Daniel H, Bornstein SS, Kane GC; Health and Public Policy Committee of the American College of Physicians. Addressing social determinants to improve patient care and promote health equity: an American College of Physicians position paper. *Ann Intern Med.* 2018;168(8):577–578 PMID: 29677265 doi: 10.7326/M17-2441
7. Committee on Integrating Social Needs Care Into the Delivery of Health Care to Improve the Nation's Health. *Integrating Social Care Into the Delivery of Health Care: Moving Upstream to Improve the Nation's Health.* National Academies of Sciences, Engineering, and Medicine; 2019
8. Schickedanz A, Hamity C, Rogers A, Sharp AL, Jackson A. Clinician experiences and attitudes regarding screening for social determinants of health in a large integrated health system. *Med Care.* 2019;57(6)(suppl 2):S197–S201 PMID: 31095061 doi: 10.1097/MLR.0000000000001051
9. Colvin JD, Bettenhausen JL, Anderson-Carpenter KD, Collie-Akers V, Chung PJ. Caregiver opinion of in-hospital screening for unmet social needs by pediatric residents. *Acad Pediatr.* 2016;16(2):161–167 PMID: 26946270 doi: 10.1016/j.acap.2015.06.002
10. Byhoff E, De Marchis EH, Hessler D, et al. Part II: a qualitative study of social risk screening acceptability in patients and caregivers. *Am J Prev Med.* 2019;57(6)(suppl 1):S38–S46 PMID: 31753278 doi: 10.1016/j.amepre.2019.07.016
11. Garg A, Brochier A, Tripodis Y, Messmer E, Drainoni ML. A social care system implemented in pediatric primary care: a cluster RCT. *Pediatrics.* 2023;152(2):e2023061513 PMID: 37492934 doi: 10.1542/peds.2023-061513
12. Gottlieb LM, Hessler D, Long D, et al. Effects of social needs screening and in-person service navigation on child health: a randomized clinical trial. *JAMA Pediatr.* 2016;170(11):e162521 PMID: 27599265 doi: 10.1001/jamapediatrics.2016.2521
13. Beck AF, Simmons JM, Sauers HS, et al. Connecting at-risk inpatient asthmatics to a community-based program to reduce home environmental risks: care system redesign using quality improvement methods. *Hosp Pediatr.* 2013;3(4):326–334 PMID: 24435190 doi: 10.1542/hpeds.2013-0047
14. Banach LP. Hospitalization: are we missing an opportunity to identify food insecurity in children? *Acad Pediatr.* 2016;16(5):438–445 PMID: 26785379 doi: 10.1016/j.acap.2016.01.002
15. Beil H, Brower HM, Chepaitis A, et al. *Accountable Health Communities (AHC) Model Evaluation: Second Evaluation Report.* Centers for Medicare & Medicaid Services; 2023. Accessed April 24, 2024. https://www.cms.gov/priorities/innovation/data-and-reports/2023/ahc-second-eval-rpt
16. Berman RS, Patel MR, Belamarich PF, Gross RS. Screening for poverty and poverty-related social determinants of health. *Pediatr Rev.* 2018;39(5):235–246 PMID: 29716966 doi: 10.1542/pir.2017-0123

17. Cartier Y, Fichtenberg F, Gottlieb L. Screening tools comparison tables. Social Interventions Research & Evaluation Network. Accessed April 24, 2024. https://sirenetwork.ucsf.edu/tools-resources/resources/screening-tools-comparison-tables
18. Systematic Review of Social Risk Screening Tools. Kaiser Permanente. Updated June 2020. Accessed April 24, 2024. https://sdh-tools-review.kpwashingtonresearch.org/find-tools
19. Narayan A, Raphael J, Rattler T, Bocchini C. *Social Determinants of Health: Screening in the Clinical Setting.* Center for Child Health Policy and Advocacy at Texas Children's Hospital; 2018
20. De Marchis EH, Brown E, Aceves B, et al. *State of the Science of Screening in Healthcare Settings.* Social Interventions Research & Evaluation Network; 2022
21. Byhoff E, LeClair AM, Smith CN, Roy TK, Drainoni ML. Designing an implementation strategy to increase health-related social needs screening: applying the PRISM framework in a resource-limited clinical setting. *Transl Behav Med.* 2023;14(3):197–205 PMID: 37897404 doi: 10.1093/tbm/ibad067
22. Friedman S, Caddle S, Motelow JE, Meyer D, Lane M. Improving screening for social determinants of health in a pediatric resident clinic: a quality improvement initiative. *Pediatr Qual Saf.* 2021;6(4):e419 PMID: 34235349 doi: 10.1097/pq9.0000000000000419
23. Mostow C, Crosson J, Gordon S, et al. Treating and precepting with RESPECT: a relational model addressing race, ethnicity, and culture in medical training. *J Gen Intern Med.* 2010;25(suppl 2):S146–S154 PMID: 20352510 doi: 10.1007/s11606-010-1274-4
24. Bouchelle Z, Bowers M, Vasan A. Ethically managing social needs data in an era of enhanced electronic health information sharing. *Pediatrics.* 2023;151(1):e2022059046 PMID: 36519251 doi: 10.1542/peds.2022-059046
25. Tyris J, Keller S, Parikh K. Social risk interventions and health care utilization for pediatric asthma: a systematic review and meta-analysis. *JAMA Pediatr.* 2022;176(2):e215103 PMID: 34870710 doi: 10.1001/jamapediatrics.2021.5103
26. The Health Leads Social Health Data Toolkit. Health Leads. Accessed April 25, 2024. https://healthleadsusa.org/news-resources/social-health-data-toolkit
27. Gottlieb L, Hessler D, Long D, Amaya A, Adler N. A randomized trial on screening for social determinants of health: the iScreen study. *Pediatrics.* 2014;134(6):e1611–e1618 PMID: 25367545 doi: 10.1542/peds.2014-1439
28. Gayle T, Law A, Stokes S, Page A, Neal W, Bhansali P. Parent preferences on screening for social determinants of health in hospitalized children. *Hosp Pediatr.* 2023;13(7):623–635 PMID: 37305961 doi: 10.1542/hpeds.2022-006718
29. Leary JC, Rijhwani L, Bettez NM, et al. Parent perspectives on screening for social needs during pediatric hospitalizations. *Hosp Pediatr.* 2022;12(8):681–690 PMID: 35843994 doi: 10.1542/hpeds.2021-006411
30. 21st Century Cures Act. US Food and Drug Administration. Accessed May 28, 2024. https://www.fda.gov/regulatory-information/selected-amendments-fdc-act/21st-century-cures-act
31. Bouchelle Z, Menko SG, Yazdani M, et al. Parent perspectives on documentation and sharing of health-related social needs data. *Hosp Pediatr.* 2024;14(4):308–316 PMID: 38477053 doi: 10.1542/hpeds.2023-007478
32. Garg A, Boynton-Jarrett R, Dworkin PH. Avoiding the unintended consequences of screening for social determinants of health. *JAMA.* 2016;316(8):813–814 PMID: 27367226 doi: 10.1001/jama.2016.9282
33. FindHelp. Accessed April 25, 2024. https://www.findhelp.org
34. About HITE. Greater New York Hospital Association. Accessed April 25, 2024. https://hitesite.org/about
35. Costich MA, Peretz PJ, Davis JA, Stockwell MS, Matiz LA. Impact of a community health worker program to support caregivers of children with special health care needs and address social determinants of health. *Clin Pediatr (Phila).* 2019;58(11–12):1315–1320 PMID: 31130003 doi: 10.1177/0009922819851263

36. Schechter SB, Lakhaney D, Peretz PJ, Matiz LA. Community health worker intervention to address social determinants of health for children hospitalized with asthma. *Hosp Pediatr.* 2021;11(12):1370–1376 PMID: 34849926 doi: 10.1542/hpeds.2021-005903

37. Klein MD, Beck AF, Henize AW, Parrish DS, Fink EE, Kahn RS. Doctors and lawyers collaborating to HeLP children—outcomes from a successful partnership between professions. *J Health Care Poor Underserved.* 2013;24(3):1063–1073 PMID: 23974381 doi: 10.1353/hpu.2013.0147

38. HEDIS MY 2023: see what's new, what's changed and what's retired. National Committee for Quality Assurance. August 1, 2022. Accessed April 25, 2024. https://www.ncqa.org/blog/hedis-my-2023-see-whats-new-whats-changed-and-whats-retired

39. Gottlieb L, DeSilvey SC, Fichtenberg C, Bernheim S, Peltz A. Developing national social care standards. *Health Affairs Forefront* blog. February 22, 2023. Accessed April 25, 2024. https://www.healthaffairs.org/content/forefront/developing-national-social-care-standards

40. Joint Commission. New requirements to reduce health care disparities. *R3 Rep.* 2022;36

41. CMS Office of Minority Health. *CMS Framework for Health Equity 2022–2032.* Centers for Medicare & Medicaid Services; 2022. Accessed April 25, 2024. https://www.cms.gov/priorities/health-equity/minority-health/equity-programs/framework

42. McQuistion K, Stokes S, Allard B, et al. Social determinants of health *ICD-10* code use in inpatient pediatrics. *Pediatrics.* 2023;152(2):e2022059319 PMID: 37431596 doi: 10.1542/peds.2022-059319

43. *CPT Evaluation and Management (E/M) Code and Guideline Changes.* American Medical Association; 2023. Accessed April 25, 2024. https://www.ama-assn.org/system/files/2023-e-m-descriptors-guidelines.pdf

44. Velasquez DE, Srinivasan S, Figueroa JF. Trends in social spending by private health insurers. *J Gen Intern Med.* 2023;38(4):1081–1083 PMID: 36357724 doi: 10.1007/s11606-022-07878-7

45. Kaiser Family Foundation. Medicaid waiver tracker: approved and pending Section 1115 waivers by state. Accessed October 1, 2024. https://www.kff.org/medicaid/issue-brief/medicaid-waiver-tracker-approved-and-pending-section-1115-waivers-by-state

Part 2. Social Drivers of Health

CHAPTER 5

Financial Assistance and Access to Care

Yonit Lax, MD, FAAP; Zoe Bouchelle, MD, MSHP, FAAP; and Aditi Vasan, MD, MSHP

Pediatric clinicians have long advocated for programs that provide families with financial assistance and support accessing health care, recognizing the potential impacts of financial need and decreased access to care on children's health and well-being. In this chapter, we introduce pediatric health care providers to local and national programs that can provide financial support and improve children's access to care. Specifically, we highlight programs that provide income support (eg, cash assistance, tax credits, employment services), address concrete resource needs (eg, nutrition programs, child care, and infant supplies), and support access to care (eg, health insurance, transportation, and internet access). We review eligibility criteria for these programs and outline practical steps providers can take to connect families to support. Finally, we discuss how pediatric providers can leverage research and patient stories to advocate for evidence-based local and national programs that reduce financial strain and bolster access to medical care for children and families.

CHAPTER 5

Financial Assistance and Access to Care

Yonit Lax, MD, FAAP; Zoe Bouchelle, MD, MSHP, FAAP; and Aditi Vasan, MD, MSHP

Introduction

As trusted partners in children's health, pediatric clinicians must consider the impact of household poverty and financial strain on child health outcomes. Financial strain is a frequent source of stress for US households, with more than a third expressing financial worry.[1] This worry is caused not only by issues related to short-term income and expenses but also by longer-term challenges related to savings, debt accumulation, and poor credit.[2] Financial strain is not equitably distributed among households in the United States as a result of years of discriminatory policies that systematically disadvantage families on the basis of their race and ethnicity, with a particularly detrimental impact on Black and Hispanic families.[3] Many policies affecting access to housing, the labor market, and financial institutions limit these families' ability to build wealth and achieve financial stability. Furthermore, evidence suggests that income and wealth inequality have continued to rise in the United States over the past several decades.[4]

A growing body of evidence suggests that poverty, income inequality, and wealth inequality are major contributors to persistent and pervasive health disparities.[5] Poverty affects children from their very first days, including their birth weight, risk of infant mortality, and early childhood development, and continues to have effects through the life course.[6] Childhood poverty can also affect brain development through exposure to toxic stress,[7] which places children experiencing poverty at increased risk for behavioral disruptions caused by poor self-regulation and executive functioning.[6] With increasing recognition of the connection between financial resources and physical health, many health care systems are beginning to incorporate social care interventions that are focused on financial strain into clinical practice. This can involve systematically screening patients and families for financial strain and connecting them to resources such as free tax preparation services, community-based organizations (CBOs), and government benefit programs that can help improve households' financial health. Addressing poverty and its impact on health may also involve addressing financial resource needs that limit access to health care, such as lack of transportation access and lack of adequate health insurance coverage. Connecting families to transportation support services and medical insurance can help ensure they have access to needed health care, and ensuring adequate insurance coverage can in turn help reduce financial strain associated with medical bills. In this chapter, we summarize key programs that provide financial assistance to families, highlight evidence on their impact, and provide practical strategies for clinicians to connect families to resources. We also highlight opportunities to advocate for anti-poverty programs and policies that can potentially improve child health and well-being.

Cash Assistance, Tax Credits, and Employment Assistance

Temporary Assistance for Needy Families

Temporary Assistance for Needy Families (TANF) is a federal program that financially assists families with low incomes. Founded in 1996, TANF not only delivers monthly cash allotments for up to 5 years but also provides other services, such as job training, education, and child care, to promote families' economic stability. Although TANF was once a major factor in protecting children from poverty, the accessibility and adequacy of TANF cash assistance have decreased dramatically since its inception.

Federal law requires that TANF cash assistance be provided only to "needy" families with children, but individual states have broad discretion to determine eligibility and benefit levels for their TANF cash assistance programs. Across all states, however, individuals must generally meet several broad requirements to be eligible, such as

- Have at least 1 child or adolescent younger than 18 years living in the household, be pregnant, or be 18 years or younger and the head of the household.
- Have a low income, usually defined as an income below a certain percentage of the federal poverty level.
- Be a US citizen or legal resident and meet other residency requirements.
- Meet education, work, or training requirements.
- Not have assets that exceed a certain amount, with this threshold determined by each state.

Since its inception, the monthly monetary value of TANF benefits has not kept pace with the rising cost of living or inflation in most states. According to data from 2021, the maximum TANF benefit for a family of 3 in every state was at or below 60% of the federal poverty level, and benefits fell below 20% of the federal poverty level in 16 states.[8] Shrinking cash benefits can limit the TANF program's ability to support families struggling to meet their basic needs.[8]

Evidence suggests that less generous TANF policies are associated with adverse health outcomes.[9] For example, research has linked more stringent TANF policies with worse parental mental health and has linked loss of TANF benefits with decreased annual preventive medical visits.[10] Although research on the benefits of TANF is mixed, TANF remains an avenue for low-income families with children to receive additional financial support in times of need.

Several states and territories have implemented innovative approaches to maximizing TANF access and participation. For example, Washington, DC, has developed integrated intake and service centers providing TANF, Supplemental Nutrition Assistance Program, Medicaid, and housing benefits so families can confirm their eligibility and complete enrollment for all these programs in one place. Pennsylvania has worked to improve the TANF programs by expanding support services, such as mental health care, transportation, child care, and housing assistance, for TANF beneficiaries and by expanding allowable education and training activities to include obtaining a high school equivalent diploma, attending community college, and attending job training programs.[11]

Supplemental Security Income and Title V Benefits

When caregivers of children with disabilities have limited income and savings, they may be eligible for monthly Supplemental Security Income (SSI) payments for their children. Children and adolescents younger than 18 years can qualify for SSI if they have a medical condition or combined conditions that meet the Social Security Administration definition of a disability. In determining eligibility for SSI and the amount of monthly SSI payments, the Social Security

Administration considers the income and resources of family members living in the child's household, the child's medical condition or combined conditions, and the expected duration of these conditions. To qualify, children must have one or more conditions that result in "marked and severe functional limitations"[12] that have been disabling or are expected to be disabling for at least 12 months. Some examples of conditions that qualify for SSI include autism, cerebral palsy, and trisomy 21 syndrome (Down syndrome). Infants born before full term or at a very low birth weight may also qualify for SSI payments, particularly in their first year after birth.

To apply for SSI, caregivers are asked to provide detailed information about their child's medical condition and how it limits their child's daily activities. They are often also asked to provide medical and school records that attest to their child's disability. State social security agencies typically take 3 to 6 months to determine whether a child meets their criteria for disability based on the information provided. For some medical conditions, however, families can receive SSI payments immediately, even as the state agency works to determine whether the child has a qualifying disability.

Once a child begins receiving SSI benefits, the Social Security Administration typically reviews their medical condition or combined conditions regularly to verify that these continue to meet eligibility criteria. This review occurs at least once every 3 years for children and adolescents younger than 18 years whose conditions are expected to improve and occurs around age 1 year for infants receiving SSI payments because of their low birth weight.

In addition to SSI benefits, many children may qualify for supplemental services through the federally funded, state-administered Maternal and Child Health Services Block Grant program, or Title V for short.[13] The federal Health Resources and Services Administration provides states with a portion of the funding needed to administer this program, and states and jurisdictions are required to match every $4 of federal Title V money they receive with at least $3 of state or local money. States use their Title V funds in a variety of ways, including working to provide care coordination, transportation support, home visiting, and nutrition counseling, with the goal of supporting the development of family-centered, community-based, coordinated systems of care.

Earned Income Tax Credit

The Earned Income Tax Credit (EITC) is a refundable tax credit that financially assists low- and moderate-income working individuals and families. Established by Congress in 1975, it was originally designed to encourage work, reduce the number of families enrolled in other welfare programs, and stimulate economic growth. It is now one of the largest and most effective anti-poverty programs in the United States.

While there have been several reforms to EITC eligibility over the past 4 decades, currently tax filers must meet 6 basic eligibility criteria:

- Have worked and earned income under a certain threshold, which varies depending on filing status and the number of qualifying children.
- Have investment income below a certain threshold.
- Have a valid Social Security number.
- Be a US citizen or US permanent resident or have a valid work visa.
- Not file for a foreign earned income exclusion.
- Have a qualifying child, who must meet certain relationship, age, and residency requirements.

In addition to eligibility reforms in the past several decades, the monetary value of the EITC has also changed with time. Currently, the amount of the EITC is based on a recipient's earned income, marital status, and number of qualifying children. The credit amount gradually decreases as income increases and phases out completely at higher income levels.

Evidence suggests that since its inception, the EITC has reduced the number of people in poverty by more than 15% and reduced child poverty by more than 25%.[14] Receipt of the EITC is associated with improved parental mental and physical health, improved birth outcomes, and improved child health, development, and educational outcomes.[15]

Child Tax Credit

The Child Tax Credit (CTC) is another tax credit designed to financially assist families with children. Established by Congress in 1997, the CTC has undergone several expansions in the intervening decades and is now a significant component of the federal government's effort to aid families with children.

To be eligible, children and adolescents must meet the following criteria:

- Be younger than age 17 years at the end of the year and meet qualifying dependent criteria.
- Provide no more than half of their own financial support during the year.
- Have lived with the filer for more than one-half of the year.
- Be properly claimed as a dependent on the tax return.
- Be a US citizen or US permanent resident or have a valid work visa.

To potentially receive the full amount of the CTC for each qualifying child, filers must meet all eligibility factors, including income.

During the height of the COVID-19 pandemic, in 2021, there was an expansion of the CTC that increased the size of the credit, expanded eligibility, made the credit fully refundable, and allowed a portion of the credit to be paid in advance monthly. Research suggests that this expansion lifted millions of children out of poverty,[16] reduced food insufficiency,[17] and was associated with reduced incidence of child abuse and neglect.[18]

Employment

Many families with children struggle financially as a result of challenges related to obtaining and maintaining consistent employment. Evidence suggests that parental job loss and long-term unemployment can have deleterious consequences for a family's poverty status, children's education attainment, and children's future employment and earnings.[19,20] In addition, income instability can have negative consequences for a child's educational attainment.[20] Clinicians may be able to mitigate some of the adverse effects of poverty on child health outcomes by helping connect families to employment support programs.

Connecting Families to Cash Assistance, Tax, and Employment Services

Key Concept

Clinicians serving low-income families and their children can play an important role in connecting these families to needed income support programs, tax preparation services, and employment assistance programs.

For TANF, eligibility and benefit levels vary by state. Clinicians can encourage families to contact their local benefits enrollment office to determine whether they qualify for TANF assistance and to learn more about their state's benefit levels and program requirements. For SSI, clinicians can make caregivers aware that their children with disabilities may be eligible for SSI. They can also provide paperwork to support these patients' SSI applications or disability reviews. For Title V benefits, clinicians can familiarize themselves with the services available through their state's Title V program, which are often listed on state Title V websites. They can then direct caregivers of children to the services and supports available through this program.

During tax season, there are several avenues for clinicians to support families in tax preparation to help ensure they claim the credits (eg, the EITC and CTC) to which they are entitled (**Table 5-1**). Clinical practice settings are increasingly implementing medical-financial partnerships (MFPs), which are cross-sector collaborations between health care organizations and financial service providers to bring financial services, including tax preparation, financial counseling, and connection to benefits, directly into clinics.[21] Clinicians can inquire about whether an MFP exists in their clinic and, if not, consider advocating to establish partnerships that increase access to financial services for families in their communities.

There are several employment support programs in the United States that are available to families with children. Examples of programs for which clinicians may refer families are included in **Table 5-2**.

In addition to making referrals to the employment support programs in **Table 5-2**, there are several other ways that clinicians can provide families with employment assistance. First, clinicians can refer families to their local social services agency to learn about available employment support programs. American Job Centers (AJCs) are an additional resource, which offer employment and training services to job seekers. Nearly 2,400 AJCs, funded by the US Department of Labor Employment and Training Administration, are located throughout the United States. Community

Table 5-1. Tax Assistance Programs

Service	How to Connect Families
Volunteer Income Tax Assistance	VITA provides free tax preparation services to individuals and families that earn approximately ≤ $60,000, people with disabilities, and taxpayers who speak a language other than English. VITA sites are typically located in public places such as community centers, libraries, and schools and are staffed by IRS-certified volunteers. The IRS provides a VITA locator tool on their website.
Internal Revenue Service Free File program	The IRS Free File program allows taxpayers who earn approximately ≤ $73,000 to use free tax preparation software provided by the IRS to prepare and file their taxes online. The software includes forms and schedules necessary for claiming tax credits such as the EITC and CTC.
MyFreeTaxes	MyFreeTaxes is an online tax preparation service provided by United Way Worldwide and H&R Block. Individuals and families of any income level can use it to file their taxes for free. Those earning less than approximately $60,000 can use the service to have their taxes prepared for them, either online or in person.
Local organizations	Many local community organizations and nonprofit groups offer free tax preparation services during tax season. Clinicians should learn about CBOs providing this resource in their area so they can refer families to these programs as needed.

Abbreviations: CBO, community-based organization; CTC, Child Tax Credit; EITC, Earned Income Tax Credit; IRS, Internal Revenue Service; VITA, Volunteer Income Tax Assistance.

Table 5-2. Employment Support Programs

Employment Support Program	Details
Temporary Assistance for Needy Families	In addition to providing cash assistance to low-income families with children, as outlined in the text, TANF provides employment services and job training to help families secure employment.
Supplemental Nutrition Assistance Program Employment and Training	SNAP E&T is a program that helps SNAP recipients gain the skills and training needed to find and maintain employment. The program provides services including job search assistance, education and training programs, and supportive services such as for transportation and child care.
Child Care and Development Fund	The CCDF provides subsidies to low-income families to help pay for child care while parents are working or in job training. States and territories administer the program, and eligibility requirements vary by state.
Early Head Start and Head Start programs	The Early Head Start and Head Start programs provide free early childhood education to low-income families with children younger than 5 years. In addition, these programs often help qualifying caregivers obtain education and employment.

Abbreviations: CCDF, Child Care and Development Fund; SNAP E&T, Supplemental Nutrition Assistance Program Employment and Training; TANF, Temporary Assistance for Needy Families.

action agencies (CAAs), which are local organizations providing services to low-income individuals, may be another helpful resource for families with employment needs. Many CAAs offer employment and training services, as well as child care assistance and other supportive services. Finally, there are several online resources that families can use to access employment support services. For example, the US Department of Labor CareerOneStop website (www.careeronestop.org) provides information on available job training programs, resources, and a directory of AJCs. State and local workforce development boards, and other state and local government websites, can also provide information on available employment support programs and services.

Nutrition Assistance, Child Care, and Infant Supplies

Nutrition Assistance

Clinicians may be able to connect low-income families to a range of government benefit programs and community-based resources that reduce financial strain. For families experiencing food insecurity, 2 key government nutrition benefit programs are the Supplemental Nutrition Assistance Program (SNAP) and the Special Supplemental Nutrition Program for Women, Infants, and Children (WIC). SNAP provides families experiencing poverty with debit cards they can use to purchase food each month.[22] About 40% of SNAP recipients live in households with one or more children, and SNAP participation has been associated with decreased rates of childhood food insecurity and improved child health.[23] WIC provides pregnant and postpartum people, infants, and children younger than 5 years with debit cards that can be used to purchase a select group of nutritious foods. WIC also provides nutrition education to these children and families and has been associated with decreased rates of low birth weight and preterm birth, decreased food insecurity, and improved nutrition.[24] But only about 50% of families that are eligible for WIC and 80% of households that are eligible for SNAP receive these benefits. Clinicians can therefore play an important role in ensuring that eligible families are aware of the WIC and SNAP programs and can receive these benefits. More information on government nutrition benefit programs is available in Chapter 7, Food Insecurity.

Child Care

Another significant expense for many low-income families is child care; many parents and caregivers struggle to find reliable and affordable child care for their children. Improving access to high-quality child care can benefit children's health and development by making it easier for parents and caregivers to obtain and maintain stable employment and by improving children's short- and long-term educational achievement.[25]

Clinicians should be aware of several programs that can provide low-cost or subsidized child care to parents with limited financial resources. The Head Start and Early Head Start programs are federally funded, state-administered programs that are available at no cost to eligible low-income families. These programs deliver child development services in center-based, home-based, or family child care settings and are designed to promote early learning and school readiness. Studies have shown that children who enroll in Head Start programs have improved social, emotional, and behavioral development and are more likely to graduate from high school and college in the future.[26]

Some states and cities also have locally funded prekindergarten programs that serve children 3 to 5 years of age and help promote kindergarten readiness. All states also provide subsidized child care to some low-income families through a federally funded, state-administered program known as the Child Care and Development Fund (CCDF). Some states also have child care tax credits that working families can use to recoup some of their child care costs.

Infant Supplies

In addition to nutrition and child care benefit programs, clinicians may be able to connect families to local clinic- or community-based resources that provide infant or child supplies, such as diapers. Research has shown that as many as 1 in 3 families in the United States report struggling to afford diapers for their children.[27] In response, more than 225 diaper banks have been built across the country. Some of these diaper banks are freestanding, whereas others were developed with or are colocated with hospitals, clinics, or social service agencies. One small pilot evaluation of a diaper bank showed that caregivers who received diapers reported improved mood, improved child health, and the ability to divert household finances toward other basic needs, such as paying for utilities and medical care.[28]

Connecting Families to Nutrition, Child Care, and Infant Supplies Services

Key Concept

Clinicians may be able to help caregivers provide essential nutrition, child care, and infant supplies for their children by connecting them to nutrition assistance programs, free or subsidized child care services, and community-based diaper banks.

For nutrition assistance, clinicians should proactively inform families about the WIC and SNAP programs and offer them assistance in enrolling in these benefit programs. Clinicians can also advocate for policy changes that streamline enrollment in WIC and SNAP, improve program retention, and make it easier for families to redeem their WIC and SNAP benefits.

For child care needs, clinicians can help families connect to Head Start or Early Head Start, locally funded prekindergarten or kindergarten programs, or their state's CCDF. In states with child care tax credits, clinicians can help make sure eligible patients' families file taxes to receive these benefits. Clinicians can also direct families in their practice to the national ChildCare.gov website or their state's Child Care Assistance Program website to learn more about the child care subsidies and free or reduced-cost child care programs that might be available in their area.

For infant supplies, clinicians can use the National Diaper Bank Network to identify community-based diaper banks in their area that may be accessible to their patients and families. Additionally, clinicians can encourage their hospitals or clinics to provide on-site diaper banks and advocate at the legislative level for existing benefit programs, such as WIC and SNAP, to incorporate on-site diaper banks at enrollment offices or distribute vouchers for subsidized diapers.

Insurance and Access to Health Care

Medicaid

Health insurance is essential for allowing families to receive needed medical care for their children, and clinicians can support families in the insurance enrollment process. About half of all children in the United States receive health insurance through their parents' or caregivers' employer-sponsored health insurance plan.[29] Children who are not eligible for insurance through a parent's or caregiver's employer may be able to receive health insurance through state-sponsored programs such as Medicaid and the Children's Health Insurance Program (CHIP) or through subsidized health plans available through state insurance exchanges.

The Medicaid program was created in 1965 as a public insurance program providing coverage for low-income individuals and families, including children, pregnant and postpartum people, and people with disabilities. More than 30 million children in low-income families across the United States currently receive Medicaid benefits. Medicaid is funded by both federal and state governments and is run at the state level, meaning each state is allowed to establish their own standards for Medicaid eligibility and benefits if they comply with certain federal guidelines. As a result, there is considerable state-level variability in Medicaid income eligibility criteria for children. Medicaid income eligibility criteria also sometimes vary by age, with higher, more generous income limits for infants younger than 1 year and lower, less generous income limits for older children. There is also considerable state-level variability in the range of services covered by Medicaid and in the accessibility of clinicians who accept Medicaid insurance, although all state Medicaid agencies are required to cover the costs of preventive care, immunizations, and dental, vision, and hearing screening for Medicaid-insured children through the Early and Periodic Screening, Diagnosis, and Treatment benefit.

Most families whose children are Medicaid insured must complete a recertification process at least once a year to ensure that their children can continue to receive Medicaid benefits. Medicaid eligibility has historically been based on monthly household income, meaning families with month-to-month income fluctuations are at risk of losing access to health insurance for their children more frequently. Because of advocacy efforts, however, beginning in January 2024 all states are required to provide 12 months of continuous eligibility for children insured by Medicaid and CHIP, meaning states will no longer be allowed to require families to recertify more than once every 12 months or to remove children from Medicaid in response to short-term income fluctuations. Some states are also exploring extended continuous eligibility to help promote access and continuity of care for children receiving Medicaid. For example, Oregon recently became the first state to allow children with Medicaid coverage to be continuously enrolled through their sixth birthday.[30] These continuous eligibility policies may help ensure access to and continuity of care.[31]

Children's Health Insurance Program

Children who are not eligible for Medicaid because their family's income falls above the program range may still be able to obtain insurance through their state CHIP program. CHIP provides free or reduced-cost health insurance coverage for children in families that do not meet income eligibility for Medicaid but may not be able to afford or obtain other forms of coverage, such as employer-sponsored or Health Insurance Marketplace insurance. Some states charge a monthly premium for CHIP coverage, but this is typically more affordable than the premium charged by analogous employer-sponsored or marketplace insurance plans and may not exceed 5% of a family's total annual income.

As with Medicaid, there is considerable state-level variability in who qualifies for CHIP, the accessibility of clinicians who accept CHIP insurance plans, and the services that CHIP covers. All state CHIP programs are required, however, to cover routine health supervision visits, immunizations, prescription medications, and hearing, dental, and vision care.

Health Insurance Exchanges

For families that do not meet income eligibility for Medicaid or CHIP and do not have employer-sponsored health insurance, another option is to obtain subsidized insurance through state health insurance exchanges. State health insurance exchanges or marketplaces are typically run by state health departments or by the federal government through Healthcare.gov. Each state Health Insurance Marketplace has an open enrollment period, which typically begins in mid-November and lasts until February, during which families can select and enroll in health plans. Health insurance exchange plans can vary widely in their premiums, deductibles, and services covered.

Access to Health Insurance for Children in Immigrant Families

Key Concept

Clinicians who care for children of immigrant families should be aware of the unique challenges these children and families might face in attempting to obtain government health insurance.

In many states, Medicaid and CHIP are not accessible to children who are undocumented immigrants or children who are legal permanent residents but have less than 5 years of permanent resident status.[32] Although several states and Washington, DC, now have state-funded programs that allow children without legal permanent resident status to enroll in either Medicaid or CHIP, more than 600,000 immigrant children across the United States remain ineligible for Medicaid and CHIP. Access to health insurance for children in immigrant families may also be limited by families' concerns about the federal "public charge" rule, which allows the US government to deny an individual's application for a visa or for legal permanent residence (a green card) if they are likely to depend on the government as their main source of financial support in the future. Current or previous use of certain government benefit programs, such as SSI and TANF, can lead applicants to be considered ineligible for a visa or for legal permanent resident status. Although Medicaid participation among children is not included in federal public charge determination and never has been, immigrant caregivers of citizen children in mixed-status households may be hesitant to seek Medicaid or CHIP coverage for these children out of fear that it will affect their own immigration status.

Transportation

Lack of access to reliable transportation directly affects access to health care and can result in missed or rescheduled appointments, delays in seeking care, and delays in following through with recommended preventive or treatment actions such as receiving vaccinations or filling prescriptions. Individuals lacking access to reliable transportation may also rely on more costly immediate care settings, such as urgent care centers or the emergency department, instead of primary care clinics, for their convenience and accessibility.

In nonurban areas, vehicle access may be particularly important because of greater transportation barriers associated with lack of public transit. Rural residents face longer travel times to seek medical care, particularly care from specialists, making vehicle access especially critical in preventing missed or delayed care. Even in urban neighborhoods, however, transportation barriers exist. Public transit routes may not align with the location of medical facilities, and unreliable service may lead to care delays. Individuals with disabilities face even greater barriers, as riding the bus or train may not be a feasible option. Transportation barriers also disproportionately affect individuals with a low income and individuals from racial and ethnic groups that have been marginalized, and as a result, these barriers can generate and perpetuate health disparities.[33] Transportation is a social determinant of health (SDOH) because of its direct influence on access to care and because of its indirect influence on other SDOH, such as employment, education, and food access.

For many families, driving, getting a ride from friends or family, or taking public transportation are all feasible modes of transportation to travel to medical appointments. Since 1966, however, Medicaid has funded nonemergency medical transportation to facilitate access to medical care for beneficiaries with disabilities who have limited public transportation access or for low-income individuals without reliable and affordable means of getting to health care appointments. State Medicaid agencies may contract with third-party organizations that coordinate transportation in return for a capitated payment, directly reimburse services, directly deliver services, or provide public transit vouchers based on geographic and individual need.[34] Although it is estimated that lack of transportation causes about 5.8 million patients in the United States to miss or delay medical care every year,[32] there is low uptake of free and subsidized medical transportation services.[35]

Improving access to medical transportation has been found to be cost effective in facilitating access to preventive services, behavioral health services, and chronic condition management for Medicaid beneficiaries.[34] More specifically, for children with asthma, the increased preventive care access and the decreased hospitalizations reduced monthly expenditures, more than offsetting increased transportation costs. One reason for low uptake of medical transportation services may be inconsistencies in how patients are screened for transportation insecurity. Screening questions vary in asking about cost, access, and impact of lack of transportation.[35]

Broadband Internet Access

In our digitally dependent world, broadband internet access is an essential resource for all families. Internet access is no longer a privilege but a basic need—providing access to school and educational resources, telemedicine, food, and job opportunities. But more than a quarter of the US population is without broadband internet access, including approximately 15% of households with school-aged children. This statistic rises to 59% among households earning less than $20,000 a year.[36]

With rising use of telemedicine, there is increasing awareness of broadband internet access as an SDOH that directly influences health outcomes. Specifically, inequitable access to telemedicine has been attributed to disparities in internet access. Further exacerbating existing health disparities seen in families that have lower incomes, that received less education, or that live in rural locations, the lack of access to the internet not only affects access to telehealth but also affects access to education, food, employment, and government benefit programs.[37]

For families experiencing financial strain, internet access may bring opportunity into their homes and improve their quality of life. Internet adoption is independently associated with improved health outcomes, a finding further supporting the claim that broadband internet access is a determinant of health that serves as a gateway to other social determinants.[38] In addition to providing health care directly, broadband internet may help facilitate access to preventive services such as public health messaging and community programming. This possibility is supported by literature showing that communities with poor access to the internet experience the highest rates of preventable hospitalizations and chronic diseases and have the lowest access to primary care.

Connecting Families to Insurance, Transportation, and Internet Services

Key Concept

Clinicians who care for low-income families can help ensure they have access to needed medical care and preventive services by informing them about the Medicaid program, assisting with enrollment paperwork, and reminding them of the need to complete recertification paperwork.

Ensuring that families can complete Medicaid recertification paperwork on time is critical to prevent temporary loss of Medicaid coverage, or "churn," which can result in gaps in needed health care despite children still being eligible for Medicaid benefits. Clinicians can also help ensure that all qualifying families have access to CHIP by referring families to their state CHIP websites, which typically include information about income guidelines as well as other enrollment requirements.

Clinicians caring for children of immigrant families should familiarize themselves with Medicaid eligibility criteria for documented and undocumented immigrants in their state and should inform caregivers of US citizen children that participating in Medicaid for their eligible children will have no bearing on their own immigration status. They may also be able to connect these families to local CBOs supporting immigrant families, which may be able to help them navigate enrollment processes and address any legal support needs.

Key Concept

Clinicians can help ensure that children have access to marketplace health insurance plans by informing families about open enrollment periods.

This may be particularly important if families are transitioning from Medicaid or CHIP to a marketplace plan or if they are moving between states, as each state has its own set of plans offered through their health insurance exchange.

Clinicians may also be able to partner with CBOs focused on health insurance and health care access to help families talk through their children's health insurance options and provide enrollment support in clinical settings. Clinicians working within larger health care organizations may also be able to refer patients to health insurance enrollment specialists employed by their health system, who may be able to directly enroll eligible patients into insurance plans. In addition, clinicians can engage in legislative advocacy focused on improving access to Medicaid, CHIP, and marketplace health insurance plans.

Key Concept

Clinicians can play an important role in supporting families' access to transportation. They can begin by screening families for unmet transportation needs and then discussing which barriers exist and whether families can see alternative clinicians to reduce transportation barriers.

Clinicians can also work with families to connect them to nonemergency medical transportation or insurance-supported transportation options. The Veterans Health Administration also offers mileage reimbursement and transportation services for some qualifying veterans and their families, and some accountable care organizations provide beneficiaries with transportation assistance in recognition of the role transportation plays as an SDOH.[33] Finally, clinicians can engage in advocacy efforts focused on encouraging their value-based payment partners, including private payers and state Medicaid agencies, to provide consistent and reliable transportation supports and services for families to reduce rates of delayed or missed medical care.

Key Concept

Clinicians can help improve broadband internet access for families in several ways. Clinicians can begin by screening families for access to the internet, working to connect them to affordable internet, and collaborating with existing community resources to create accessibility for families at a local level.

Launched in 2021, the Affordable Connectivity Program, a US government program run by the Federal Communications Commission (www.affordableconnectivity.gov) is one resource that was created for families struggling to afford internet access. The Affordable Connectivity Program provides a $30-per-month discount on internet service for qualifying households ($75-per-month on Native lands). Families are eligible if household income is below 200% of the federal poverty level or if a household member receives a government benefit such as SNAP, Medicaid, SSI, WIC, a Pell Grant, or free and reduced-price lunches. In addition to discounted internet service, individuals may qualify for up to $100 toward purchasing a computer or device to access the internet. Locally, many communities are also working toward achieving digital equity through the creation of low-cost Wi-Fi hot spots and internet access provided at public libraries and community centers.[39] Finally, clinicians can advocate for local governments to provide portable hot spots and put digital equity on their advocacy agendas.

Conclusion

As trusted partners in children's health, clinicians must consider the impact of household financial strain on child health outcomes and work to mitigate this strain for families in our clinical practice. Many of us can recall patients whose health was directly affected by their families' financial strain, including infants who missed essential health supervision visits and vaccinations because their families were unable to afford transportation, children with asthma who experienced acute exacerbations because their families lost insurance coverage and could not afford to pay for their medications out of pocket, and families that could not complete telehealth appointments because they had limited or inconsistent access to broadband internet. Understanding the landscape of programs that provide financial assistance, transportation assistance, and health insurance coverage in the United States may help clinicians advocate for their patients by answering their questions and by facilitating access to the resources and supports they need.

With the knowledge gained from this chapter, it is our hope that clinicians will also consider advocating on a community level, partnering with CBOs already working in these areas to integrate services into clinical care, or working together with these organizations through direct referrals, ideally with closed-loop communication. And on a legislative level, clinicians should consider leveraging their expertise in children's health and their experiences caring for families with financial strain to advocate for policy changes that improve access to and funding for government benefit programs that address financial strain and reduce barriers to health care for low-income families and their children.

Key Points

- Poverty, income inequality, and wealth inequality are major contributors to adverse child health outcomes and child health disparities.
- Clinicians should understand the landscape of programs that provide financial assistance, transportation assistance, and health insurance coverage in the United States so they can support families in need to connect to available resources.
- Key financial assistance programs include cash assistance, tax credits, and employment assistance.
- Key programs that assist with concrete resource needs include government nutrition benefit programs such as WIC and SNAP, child care assistance programs, and diaper banks.
- Key programs that can support health care access include health insurance programs like Medicaid, CHIP, and subsidized insurance plans available through state exchanges; subsidized medical transportation programs; and programs focused on expanding broadband internet access.
- Clinicians may also have the opportunity to promote improved child health and well-being by using their trusted voices to advocate for the implementation and expansion of anti-poverty programs and policies.

References

1. Stress in America: money, inflation, war pile on to nation stuck in COVID-19 survival mode. News release. American Psychological Association; March 11, 2022. Accessed May 1, 2024. https://www.apa.org/news/press/releases/stress/2022/march-2022-survival-mode?utm_source=twitter&utm_medium=social&utm_campaign=apa-stress&utm_content=sia-mar22-money#inflation
2. Ryu S, Fan L. The relationship between financial worries and psychological distress among U.S. adults. *J Fam Econ Issues*. 2023;44(1):16–33 PMID: 35125855 doi: 10.1007/s10834-022-09820-9
3. Bowdler J, Harris B. Racial inequality in the United States. US Department of the Treasury. July 21, 2022. Accessed May 1, 2024. https://home.treasury.gov/news/featured-stories/racial-inequality-in-the-united-states#_ftn8
4. Kent AH, Ricketts LR. Has wealth inequality in America changed over time? here are key statistics. Federal Reserve Bank of St Louis. December 2, 2020. Accessed August 8, 2023. https://www.stlouisfed.org/open-vault/2020/december/has-wealth-inequality-changed-over-time-key-statistics
5. Oberg C, Colianni S, King-Schultz L. Child health disparities in the 21st century. *Curr Probl Pediatr Adolesc Health Care*. 2016;46(9):291–312 PMID: 27712646 doi: 10.1016/j.cppeds.2016.07.001
6. Duffee J, Kuo A, Gitterman B; American Academy of Pediatrics Council on Community Pediatrics. Poverty and child health in the United States. *Pediatrics*. 2016;137(4):e20160339 PMID: 26962238 doi: 10.1542/peds.2016-0339
7. Garner AS, Shonkoff JP, Earls MF, et al; American Academy of Pediatrics Section on Developmental and Behavioral Pediatrics. Early childhood adversity, toxic stress, and the role of the pediatrician: translating developmental science into lifelong health. *Pediatrics*. 2012;129(1):e224–e231 PMID: 22201148 doi: 10.1542/peds.2011-2662
8. Thompson GA, Azevedo-McCaffrey D, Carr D. Increases in TANF cash benefit levels are critical to help families meet rising costs. Center on Budget and Policy Priorities. Updated February 3, 2023. Accessed May 1, 2024. https://www.cbpp.org/research/family-income-support/more-states-raising-tanf-benefits-to-boost-families-economic-security

9. Finkelstein DM, Harding JF, Paulsell D, English B, Hijjawi GR, Ng'andu J. Economic well-being and health: the role of income support programs in promoting health and advancing health equity. *Health Aff (Millwood)*. 2022;41(12):1700–1706 PMID: 36469819 doi: 10.1377/hlthaff.2022.00846

10. Narain K, Ettner S. The impact of exceeding TANF time limits on the access to healthcare of low-income mothers. *Soc Work Public Health*. 2017;32(7):452–460 PMID: 28816637 doi: 10.1080/19371918.2017.1360817

11. Rodrigue S, Lyons M, Nelson M. Seven ways to improve TANF and help families advance. American Public Human Services Association. August 22, 2022. Accessed May 1, 2024. https://aphsa.org/APHSABlog/TANF-modernization-22/seven-ways-to-improve-TANF-and-help-families.aspx

12. Social Security Administration. Understanding Supplemental Security Income SSI for Children—2024 Edition. Accessed June 12, 2024. https://www.ssa.gov/ssi/text-child-ussi.htm

13. Title V Maternal and Child Health (MCH) Services Block Grant. Health Resources and Services Administration Maternal and Child Health Bureau. December 2023. Accessed May 1, 2024. https://mchb.hrsa.gov/programs-impact/title-v-maternal-child-health-mch-block-grant

14. Nichols A, Rothstein J. The Earned Income Tax Credit. In: Moffitt RA, ed. *Economics of Means-Tested Transfer Programs in the United States*. Vol 1. University of Chicago Press; 2016:chap2

15. Simon D, McInerney M, Goodell S. The Earned Income Tax Credit, poverty, and health. *Health Aff Health Policy Brief*. 2018 doi: 10.1377/hpb20180817.769687

16. Parolin Z, Collyer S, Curran MA, Wimer C. Monthly poverty rates among children after the expansion of the Child Tax Credit. Center on Poverty and Social Policy. August 20, 2021. Accessed May 1, 2024. https://static1.squarespace.com/static/610831a16c95260dbd68934a/t/6125831bb2d0cb07e98375b9/1629848348974/Monthly-Poverty-with-CTC-July-CPSP-2021.pdf

17. Shafer PR, Gutiérrez KM, Ettinger de Cuba S, Bovell-Ammon A, Raifman J. Association of the implementation of Child Tax Credit advance payments with food insufficiency in US households. *JAMA Netw Open*. 2022;5(1):e2143296 PMID: 35024837 doi: 10.1001/jamanetworkopen.2021.43296

18. Bullinger LR, Boy A. Association of expanded Child Tax Credit payments with child abuse and neglect emergency department visits. *JAMA Netw Open*. 2023;6(2):e2255639 PMID: 36795416 doi: 10.1001/jamanetworkopen.2022.55639

19. Coelli MB. Parental job loss and the education enrollment of youth. *Labour Econ*. 2011;18(1):25–35 doi: 10.1016/j.labeco.2010.04.015

20. Hardy BL. Childhood income volatility and adult outcomes. *Demography*. 2014;51(5):1641–1665 PMID: 25280839 doi: 10.1007/s13524-014-0329-2

21. Marcil LE, Barnett KG, Zuckerman B. Medical–financial partnerships—beyond traditional boundaries. *N Engl J Med*. 2021;385(4):289–291 PMID: 34279067 doi: 10.1056/NEJMp2101731

22. *A Quick Guide to SNAP Eligibility and Benefits*. Center on Budget and Policy Priorities; 2023. Accessed May 2, 2024. https://www.cbpp.org/research/food-assistance/a-quick-guide-to-snap-eligibility-and-benefits

23. Food and Nutrition Service. Yearly trends SNAP households by demographic and income characteristics. US Department of Agriculture. Accessed May 2, 2024. https://www.fns.usda.gov/SNAP-household-trends

24. Hamad R, Collin DF, Baer RJ, Jelliffe-Pawlowski LL. Association of revised WIC food package with perinatal and birth outcomes: a quasi-experimental study. *JAMA Pediatr*. 2019;173(9):845–852 PMID: 31260072 doi: 10.1001/jamapediatrics.2019.1706

25. Morrissey TW. Child care and parent labor force participation: a review of the research literature. *Rev Econ Househ*. 2017;15(1):1–24 doi: 10.1007/s11150-016-9331-3

26. Head Start services. Office of Head Start. Updated June 30, 2023. Accessed May 2, 2024. https://www.acf.hhs.gov/ohs/about/head-start

27. Smith MV, Kruse A, Weir A, Goldblum J. Diaper need and its impact on child health. *Pediatrics.* 2013;132(2):253–259 PMID: 23897910 doi: 10.1542/peds.2013-0597

28. Massengale KEC, Erausquin JT, Old M. Health, social, and economic outcomes experienced by families as a result of receiving assistance from a community-based diaper bank. *Matern Child Health J.* 2017;21(10):1985–1994 PMID: 28710698 doi: 10.1007/s10995-017-2317-9

29. Health insurance coverage of children 0-18. Kaiser Family Foundation. Accessed May 2, 2024. https://www.kff.org/other/state-indicator/children-0-18/?currentTimeframe=0&sortModel=%7B%22colId%22:%22Location%22,%22sort%22:%22asc%22%7D#

30. Alker J, Burak EW. Oregon leads the nation by covering children in Medicaid from birth to kindergarten—which state will be next?? Center for Children and Families at the McCourt School of Public Policy. September 28, 2022. Accessed May 2, 2024. https://ccf.georgetown.edu/2022/09/28/oregon-leads-the-nation-by-covering-children-in-medicaid-from-birth-to-kindergarten-which-state-will-be-next

31. Vasan A, Kenyon CC, Fiks AG, Venkataramani AS. Continuous eligibility and coverage policies expanded children's Medicaid enrollment. *Health Aff (Millwood).* 2023;42(6):753–758 PMID: 37276479 doi: 10.1377/hlthaff.2022.01465

32. Lacarte V. Immigrant children's Medicaid and CHIP access and participation: a data profile. Migration Policy Institute. June 2022. Accessed May 2, 2024. https://www.migrationpolicy.org/research/immigrant-children-medicaid-chip

33. Wolfe MK, McDonald NC, Holmes MG. Transportation barriers to health care in the United States: findings from the National Health Interview Survey, 1997–2017. *Am J Public Health.* 2020;110(6):815–822 PMID: 32298170 doi: 10.2105/AJPH.2020.305579

34. Musumeci M, Rudowitz R. Medicaid non-emergency medical transportation: overview and key issues in Medicaid expansion waivers. Kaiser Family Foundation. February 24, 2016. Accessed May 2, 2024. https://www.kff.org/medicaid/issue-brief/medicaid-non-emergency-medical-transportation-overview-and-key-issues-in-medicaid-expansion-waivers

35. Razon N, Gottlieb L. Content analysis of transportation screening questions in social risk assessment tools: are we capturing transportation insecurity? *J Am Board Fam Med.* 2022;35(2):400–405 PMID: 35379729 doi: 10.3122/jabfm.2022.02.210256

36. Vogels EA, Perrin A, Rainie L, Anderson M. 53% of Americans say the internet has been essential during the COVID-19 outbreak. Pew Research Center. April 30, 2020. Accessed May 2, 2024. https://www.pewresearch.org/internet/2020/04/30/53-of-americans-say-the-internet-has-been-essential-during-the-covid-19-outbreak

37. Benda NC, Veinot TC, Sieck CJ, Ancker JS. Broadband internet access is a social determinant of health! *Am J Public Health.* 2020;110(8):1123–1125 PMID: 32639914 doi: 10.2105/AJPH.2020.305784

38. Federal Communications Commission. Studies and data analytics on broadband and health. Accessed May 2, 2024. https://www.fcc.gov/health/sdoh/studies-and-data-analytics

39. Ortega G, Rodriguez JA, Maurer LR, et al. Telemedicine, COVID-19, and disparities: policy implications. *Health Policy Technol.* 2020;9(3):368–371 PMID: 32837888 doi: 10.1016/j.hlpt.2020.08.001

CHAPTER 6

Housing as a Driver of Health

Marc F. Shi, MD, MSc

Access to safe, affordable, stable housing has long been recognized as a key determinant of physical and mental health. Unfortunately, this resource is out of reach for many US residents. In addition to the failure of new housing stock being made available to meet increasing demands, costs of housing—for both renters and homeowners—continues to rise across the country. The most distal outcome of this continuation is an increase in homelessness, which is particularly concerning given the myriad negative health effects of being unhoused. These worrying trends are not a new phenomenon and do not affect all communities equally. By examining historical precedents for our current crisis, including racially discriminatory housing policy and stagnating support of our public housing infrastructure, we can identify how we arrived at our current state of affordable housing and how communities of color and communities with low incomes have come to be disproportionately harmed.

CHAPTER 6

Housing as a Driver of Health

Marc F. Shi, MD, MSc

Introduction

The health effects of increasing housing costs and decreasing access are manifold but can be conceptualized into 4 key pathways: housing quality/conditions, housing affordability/cost, housing stability/insecurity, and neighborhood effects. Given the growing evidence supporting how each of these pathways influence housing outcomes, there are increasing efforts to identify and address housing needs in clinical settings. Housing quality and stability issues have shown to be reliably identifiable in both primary care and immediate care environments, and there are ongoing efforts to effectively implement these screening tools into regular practice. Similarly, various models to address housing needs in health care are currently being studied. These range from integration of community health workers (CHWs) into practice settings as a specialized ancillary workforce to address needs as they arise to interprofessional partnerships such as medical-legal clinics. While there are barriers to effectively implementing and replicating these interventions, the centrality of safe, stable housing in health outcomes means that it is increasingly a priority for both health care professionals and health systems to meet the housing needs of their patients and communities as part of a comprehensive approach to health.

State of Housing in the United States

Housing costs continue to rise, and housing stock fails to keep pace, particularly for those facing significant socioeconomic barriers. This section discusses imbalances between growth of the national housing stock and need for affordable housing as well as how that imbalance contributes to a growing crisis of homelessness and housing instability across the country.

Housing Stock

It is increasingly difficult for families to find safe, stable, affordable housing. According to the Harvard Joint Center for Housing Studies (JCHS),[1] the total number of people paying rent in the United States (subsequently referred to as *renters*) has been steadily growing, with an increase of more than 870,000 from the first quarter of 2020 to the third quarter of 2021. This demand has far outpaced supply, with 611,000 apartments becoming newly occupied during this period and only 250,000 new vacant units completing construction. As expected, this imbalance between available housing stock and demand hits households with low incomes the hardest. The National Low Income Housing Coalition (NLIHC) annually assesses the availability of housing stock for low-income households.[1,2] Using the income thresholds defined in **Box 6-1**, the 2022 NLIHC

Box 6-1.
Definitions of Area Median Income and Income Eligibility Brackets as Determined by the US Department of Housing and Urban Development

Area median income: Calculated by HUD annually, is a measure of the median income for a household in a predefined geographic region, primarily based on a metropolitan statistical area. A household with an income meeting AMI would be at "100% AMI."

Extremely low income: Household income <30% of AMI or the federal poverty guideline.

Very low income: Household income 31%–50% of AMI.

Low income: Household income 51%–80% of AMI.

Abbreviations: AMI, area median income; HUD, US Department of Housing and Urban Development.

report shows that 11 million renter households are considered to have extremely low incomes (ELIs), making up approximately 25% of all US renting households. Of those households, Black and Latine populations are more likely to be renting and more likely to be considered to have ELIs. For example, 57% of Black households are renters and 19% of households have ELIs compared to 19% of white households that are renters and 6% that have ELIs. The NLIHC further found that no state has an adequate supply of rental housing for ELI renters, with a range from 18 to 61 homes for every 100 ELI renters across all 50 states.

Cost of Housing

In addition to there being a limited supply of affordable housing, renters are facing significant increases in the cost of housing. A household is *rent burdened,* as defined by the US Department of Housing and Urban Development (HUD), when it spends more than 30% of household income on rent and *severely rent burdened* when it spends more than 50% of household income on rent. Drawing on American Community Survey data, the Harvard JCHS in 2021 saw an all-time high in rent burden across the country, with more than 21 million households (approximately 49% of all renters in the country) experiencing rent burden, the highest in 20 years of data collection (**Figure 6-1**). This held true across all incomes and was attributed to changes in renter incomes during the COVID-19 pandemic. Homeowners also experienced increased burden during this time, with 22.8% of them—approximately 19 million households—spending more than 30% of their income on housing.

State of Homelessness

Perhaps the most urgent outcome of these alarming trends in housing access and affordability is the growing number of households that are unable to maintain a stable place to live. Although public perceptions of homelessness often center on the segment of the population that experiences chronic homelessness (ie, individuals without stable housing for >1 year), the state of homelessness is, in fact, much more fluid, and many more individuals experience transient homelessness for short periods. As such, it is difficult to fully capture the range of circumstances into which people experiencing homelessness are placed. For analytic and policy purposes, HUD provides a standard definition of homelessness used by most local governments and agencies (**Box 6-2**).

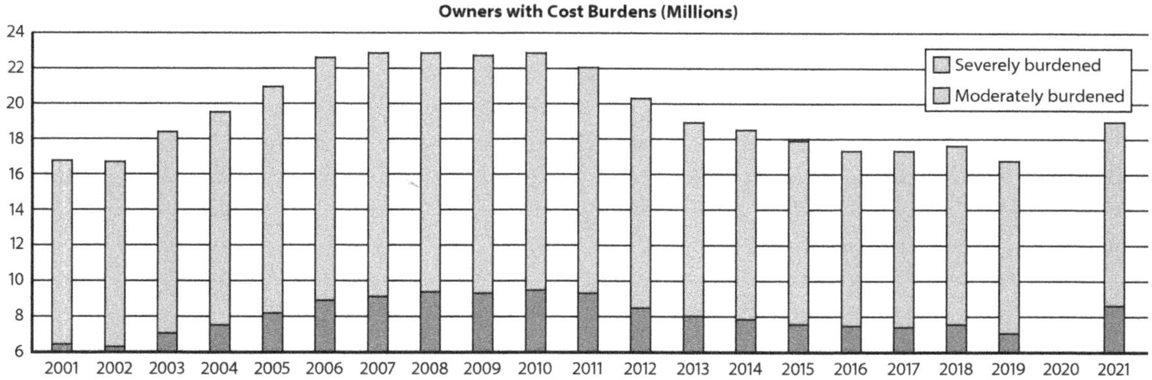

Figure 6-1. Trends in Proportion of Homeowners Experiencing Cost Burden

Harvard Joint Center for Housing Studies tabulation of American Community Survey data showing trends in rent burden experienced nationally.

From Whitney P. Number of renters burdened by housing costs reached a record high in 2021. Harvard Joint Center for Housing Studies. February 1, 2023. Accessed May 3, 2024. https://www.jchs.harvard.edu/blog/number-renters-burdened-housing-costs-reached-record-high-2021.

Box 6-2.

US Department of Housing and Urban Development Definition of *Homelessness*

"(1) Individuals and families who lack a fixed, regular, and adequate nighttime residence and includes a subset for an individual who resided in an emergency shelter or a place not meant for human habitation and who is exiting an institution where he or she temporarily resided; (2) individuals and families who will imminently lose their primary nighttime residence; (3) unaccompanied youth and families with children and youth who are defined as homeless under other federal statutes who do not otherwise qualify as homeless under this definition; and (4) individuals and families who are fleeing, or are attempting to flee, domestic violence, dating violence, sexual assault, stalking, or other dangerous or life-threatening conditions that relate to violence against the individual or a family member."

Further clarification to this defines *youth* as younger than 25 years and *shelter* as "emergency shelter" but not "transitional housing."

Reproduced in part from HUD's definition of homelessness: resources and guidance. HUD Exchange. March 8, 2019. Accessed May 3, 2024. https://www.hudexchange.info/news/huds-definition-of-homelessness-resources-and-guidance.

Using this definition, HUD conducts its annual Point-in-Time Count, a nationwide homelessness census done on a single night of the year (typically in January), including people living in shelters, people living in transitional housing, and people living unsheltered. For example, in 2022, the count revealed a total of 582,462 individuals with circumstances meeting the definition of homelessness. This is a significant increase from the total of 380,657 in 2021. It has been attributed to growing economic stressors in the setting of the COVID-19 pandemic as well as changes in the count during the early years of the pandemic itself. Chronic homelessness in

2022 saw an increase of 15.5% from 2020 and an increase of 20.4% from 2010. The Point-in-Time Count itself is often criticized for likely underestimating the total number of people experiencing unstable housing, as it often misses large numbers of people who are in health care settings such as emergency departments (EDs), who may be doubling up with relatives, or who are otherwise in unstable but sheltered environments. Finally, there are notable racial and ethnic disparities in who is affected by homelessness. Black people make up 37% of homeless populations compared to 12% of the total US population; there has also been an 8% increase in Latine individuals experiencing homelessness from 2020 to 2022.

Key Concept

It is increasingly difficult to find housing at all, let alone housing that is affordable and safe. This has been the case for years and only dramatically worsened during the COVID-19 pandemic. Because of this trend, homelessness has seen a significant increase in recent years. Although the impacts of this are widespread, they disproportionately affect communities of color with low incomes.

Root Causes of the Housing Crisis

The current housing crisis is not without precedent. The barriers that families in poverty encounter, particularly families that have been racially and ethnically marginalized, to find safe, affordable housing can be seen as an extension of decades-old policies restricting access to housing to certain populations.

Racism and Housing

In the United States, there is evidence that racism and exclusion have been and still are deeply embedded within the option for certain individuals and communities to obtain property. Policy and practice, both formal and informal, have systematically excluded oppressed populations from obtaining housing—namely, individuals and families of color (**Box 6-3**).

Attempts by the federal government to preserve and bolster homeownership for families struggling during the Great Depression led to the creation of the Home Owners' Loan Corporation in 1933 and the Federal Housing Administration in 1934.[3] These agencies used risk assessments to determine approval for their loans, and both used racial composition as a factor in these assessments: neighborhoods with high proportions of Black families were consistently considered "high risk."[4] The term *redlining* refers to how these neighborhoods were demarcated with a "red line" indicating risk, thus excluding them from loan support (**Figure 6-2**).[5] The exclusion of Black families from these stable, lower-interest loans meant both overall lower rates of homeownership and higher usage of risky, high-interest loans that were more prone to default and foreclosure. Today, maps of areas that have been historically redlined have been shown to

Box 6-3.

Examples of Legislation and Practices Exacerbating Residential Racial Segregation

Numerous practices have existed (and still exist) that make it disproportionately difficult for certain communities to obtain stable, affordable housing, such as

- **Redlining:** Practice by which federal mortgage loans were denied to families in majority-Black neighborhoods based on racialized assessments of risk.
- **Racial covenants:** Formal and informal agreements among local communities to exclude primarily Black families from homeownership within certain neighborhoods.
- **Exclusionary zoning:** Use of seemingly race-neutral features, such as density, to maintain racial and socioeconomic segregation.

correspond to current areas of social vulnerability, including increased susceptibility to disasters and disease outbreaks[6] and, more recently, COVID-19 incidence rates,[7] illustrating the way in which these exclusionary policies resonate today.

Black families were also often restricted from buying or renting homes through informal means. Records from deeds from the 19th through the early 20th century explicitly forbid the sale to Black households, and increasingly through the 20th century, white neighborhoods and neighborhood associations made informal compacts, or covenants, to prevent sales to Black families.[3] These practices were tacitly unopposed or explicitly supported by government at all levels.[8] The racial exclusionary language in covenants was not deemed unlawful until the Fair Housing Act of 1968.[3,4]

Even without explicitly racist language, other forms of exclusion de facto barred people of color from living in certain neighborhoods. Zoning laws that allowed only certain types of construction (eg, single-family homes and not multifamily homes, density-based zoning) in certain (predominantly white) areas limited the types of housing options available in those areas, thus preventing families in poverty and families of color from living in well-resourced neighborhoods.[9–11] Exclusionary zoning such as this persisted in various forms and even exists to this day, both restricting the development of diverse housing options and preventing the movement of individuals, largely families in poverty and families of color.[12]

Decline of Public Housing and Growth of the Private Real Estate Industry

Compounding barriers to finding safe, affordable housing in the private market is the inadequate supply of public housing. The Housing Act of 1937 was the first attempt by the US government to support the actual provision of housing, providing funding to local housing authorities to build and maintain public housing units for US residents. By the 1970s and 1980s, policies of austerity led to a moratorium on public housing funding and construction under the Nixon administration,[13] and disinvestment in existing housing led to worsening quality and disrepair.[13–15]

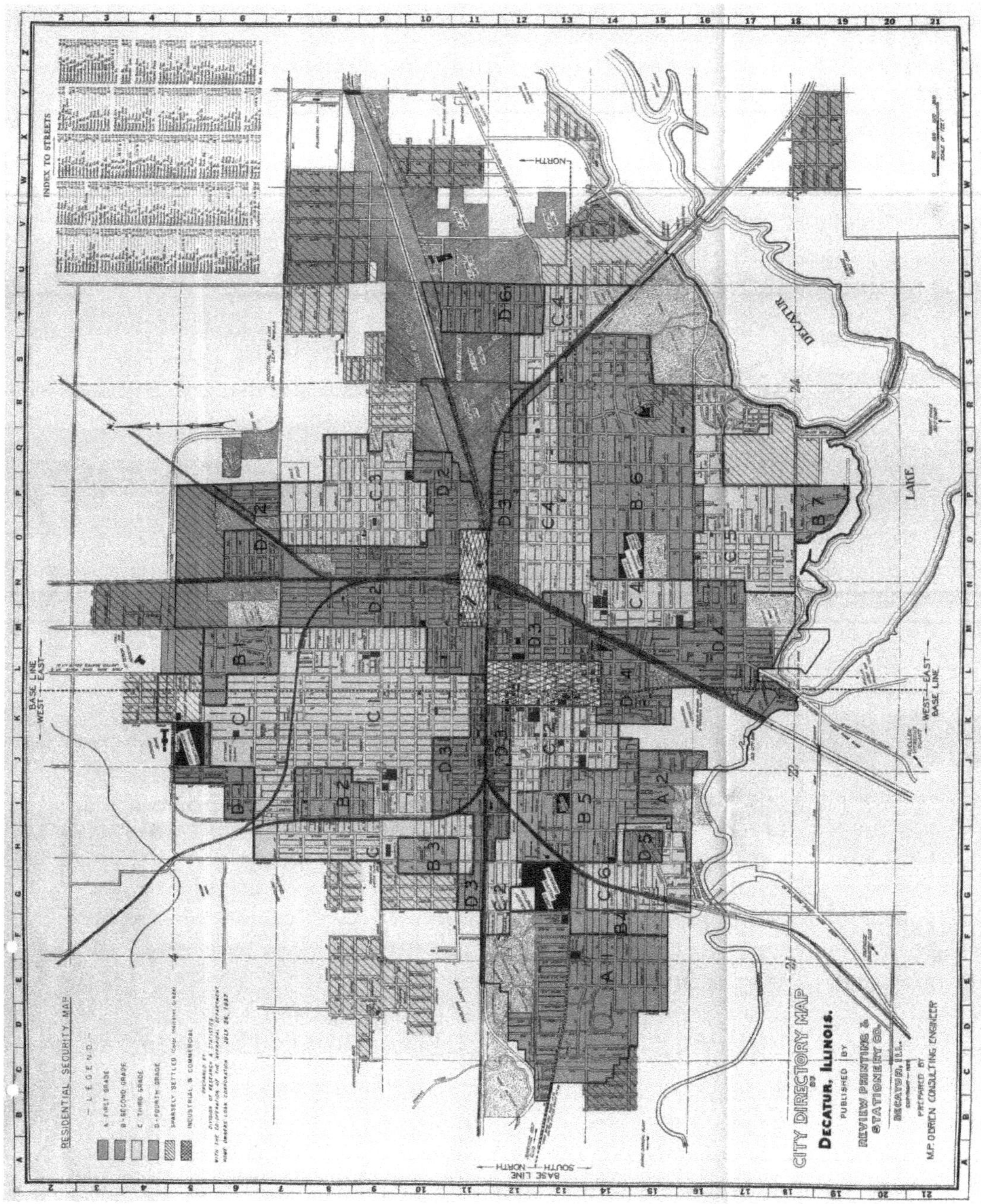

Figure 6-2. Redlining Map of Decatur, IL

Reproduced from Nelson RK, Madron J, Champine R, Devers C, et al. *Mapping Inequality: Redlining in New Deal America.* University of Richmond. Accessed May 3, 2024. https://dsl.richmond.edu/panorama/redlining.

Key Concept

There are numerous historical antecedents to our current housing crisis. In particular, historical policies lay the groundwork for today's pattern of racial segregation and racial disparities in housing and the lack of available housing options for those most impacted by poverty.

Parallel with the decline of public housing has been the growth of the real estate industry. Private real estate and development are a dominant force in both the United States and global economies; a report from real estate tracker Redfin shows that investors owned the largest share of homes in the fourth quarter of 2021, with a total value of $50 billion.[16] Private equity companies are also increasingly playing a role,[17] with the investment firm Blackstone being the largest owner of commercial real estate in the world.[18] Although some point to the need for private developers and real estate to fund increases in housing stock, numerous efforts across the country by community organizers and advocates now call for a reevaluation of our housing infrastructure that questions the reliance on profit-driven development.[19]

Impact of Housing on Health: 4 Key Mechanisms

A large and growing body of literature has identified the ways in which housing can affect the health of individuals and communities. This effect has been conceptualized as working through 4 interrelated mechanisms: housing quality/conditions, housing affordability/cost, housing stability/insecurity and neighborhood effects (**Figure 6-3**).[20] Exploring each of these mechanisms in turn allows for a view of the multifaceted ways in which housing affects health.

Housing Quality/Conditions

A significant portion of the literature centers on how the physical conditions of one's housing affects health.[21] Housing quality's effect on health can be further characterized as the structural condition of the housing itself, housing as protection from other environmental hazards, and harmful exposures from inadequate and poor-quality housing.

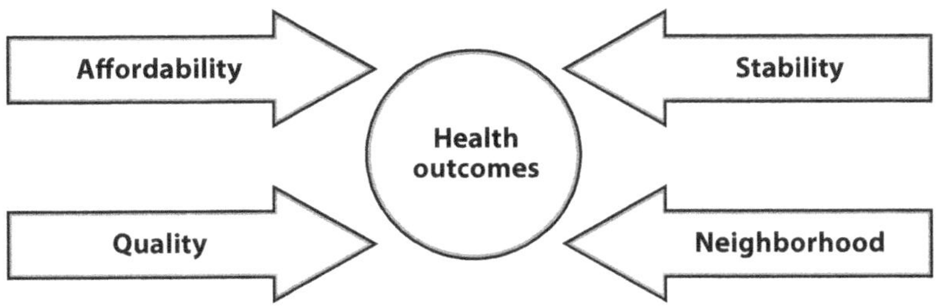

Figure 6-3. Four Key Mechanisms of Housing That Affect Health

Adapted with permission from Taylor L. Housing and health: an overview of the literature. *Health Aff Policy Brief.* June 7, 2018. Accessed October 17, 2024. https://www.healthaffairs.org/content/briefs/housing-and-health-overview-literature.

Toxic Exposures

Perhaps the most widely recognized hazard from unsafe building materials is lead exposure, which is associated with a variety of neurological and cognitive effects that persist throughout the life span, and the risk is present with even low levels of exposure (**Box 6-4**). Exposure in the home, specifically to lead paint, is the most common cause of lead exposure, and the highest risk exists among infants and children between 1 and 6 years old. Since lead paint was banned after 1978, the risk is highest in older housing, and given that much of the country's low-income and public housing stock is older and less frequently refurbished, this risk is highest among families in poverty with fewer housing options.[22–24] Thankfully, since the ban on lead in housing materials, there have been efforts at all levels of government to retrofit and rehabilitate older buildings to mitigate lead exposure, resulting in reduced overall lead exposure.

In addition to toxic building materials, there are numerous other household irritants that can affect health. Within the home, exposure to pest allergens (eg, rodents, cockroaches) is associated with worsening respiratory disease, particularly childhood asthma.[25] Early childhood exposure to allergens and ongoing exposure has been associated with the development and continuation of sensitization and airway inflammation.[26] Racial disparities have also been noted to be associated with these effects. Asthma prevalence is disproportionately high among Black and Latine children and low-income children; similarly, exposure to poor housing conditions, mold, and indoor allergens is disproportionately high for these communities. Studies in multiple communities across the country[27,28] suggest that the poor housing conditions disproportionately experienced by communities of color likely contribute to increased rates of household irritants and, thereby, childhood respiratory disease.

Safety, Injuries, and Structural Stability

According to World Health Organization estimates, injuries in the home account for approximately one-third of all injuries globally and, as a portion of unintentional injuries overall, are likely to significantly contribute to morbidity nationally and globally.[29] Such injuries include falls, burns, poisoning, smoke inhalation, cuts, drownings, or being crushed or hit from collapsing buildings. Of these, falls make up the largest proportion of injuries requiring medical attention. Although falls are often thought of in the context of individual risk (eg, medical conditions predisposing a person to falls, weakness, gait) or local home environment (eg, rugs, wires, stairs), structural stability and conditions of housing play a large role in mediating risk for falls. For example, features of housing related to fall risk include uneven floors, inadequate lighting, uneven stairs or stairs without handrails, and windows without child locks or guards.

Box 6-4.
Lead Exposure Risk Assessment

Current American Academy of Pediatrics guidelines recommend risk assessment for lead exposure at **6, 9, 12, 18, and 24 months of age and at 3, 4, 5, and 6 years of age.** Blood lead level testing is recommended **only** if the risk assessment is concerning.

Derived from Hagan JF Jr, Shaw JS, Duncan PM, eds. *Bright Futures: Guidelines for Health Supervision of Infants, Children, and Adolescents.* 4th ed. American Academy of Pediatrics; 2017.

Heating and Cooling

Climate change has led to shifting temperatures and weather conditions across the entire United States. This has also led to increasing attention to the risks of heat and cold exposure. The ability to regulate temperature inside one's residence is a clear factor in mediating the risks of these environmental exposures. Existing observational and some experimental data support this finding. In Detroit, MI, a community survey showed an association between the lack of air-conditioning and the odds of heat-related hazards.[30] In a large epidemiological study in the United Kingdom, the inability to protect against cold weather was also associated with an increased use of health services.[31] Similarly, interventions to improve heating and cooling conditions in houses have shown positive effects on self-reported health and use of health services. For example, a cluster randomized trial of implementing insulation in existing homes improved heating in the home, reduced days of fair/poor self-reported health, and reduced days of wheezing, off work, or off school. It also led to a statistically nonsignificant trend in reduced ED visits.[32] A large 2013 Cochrane Review of interventions on housing conditions to improve health, despite mixed findings, showed that interventions addressing warmth and heating and building conditions showed the strongest consistent findings in improving respiratory health and mental health outcomes.[33]

Unfortunately, for many families, the ability to regularly maintain appropriate heating and cooling can be a significant financial burden. A 2020 report from the American Council for an Energy-Efficient Economy showed that, nationally, lower-income households spent 8.1% of their income on energy costs, as opposed to 2.3% for higher-income households, and a quarter of lower-income households have energy cost burdens of more than 14.4%.[34] Racial disparities also exist in the distribution of this burden: the median energy burden on Black households is 45% higher than on non-Hispanic white households.

As such, it would also follow that providing support for stable utilities is an important piece of preventing health harms. National programs such as the Low Income Home Energy Assistance Program (LIHEAP), created in 1981, financially assist low-income households. The evidence suggests that such programs, by decreasing the burden of energy costs and maintaining utilities, can support health. Data from the national LIHEAP show that families enrolled in this program experience a lower risk for evident undernutrition and a lower risk for hospitalization.[35]

Key Concept

The physical properties of one's housing, from the materials used in its construction; its ability to shield inhabitants from environmental exposure; or the harmful exposures associated with poor housing can all affect an individual's health.

Clinicians can support patients facing housing quality issues by

- **Assessing for harmful exposures, especially in patients with associated chronic illness (eg, asthma)**
- **Referring to local programs focused on addressing relevant health hazards (eg, lead abatement programs, air pollutant programs)**
- **Identifying and referring patients to local and national programs that subsidize costs of utilities or address housing-related hazards (eg, LIHEAP)**

Housing Affordability/Cost

Growing data show that the high-cost burden for housing leads to trade-offs that negatively affect health. For example, a family with an income of $2,000 per month, paying fair market rent (40th percentile market rent for standard quality units) of $1,295, has only $705 remaining for all other nonhousing expenses. This would inevitably lead the family to make trade-offs in deciding how to distribute those funds, for example, forgoing medical visits to pay for food. People living in unaffordable housing had increased odds of self-reported poor health, as well as increased cost-related health care engagement and medication taking.[36,37] Housing instability, which may result from high rental costs, has also been associated with delayed access to care, delayed prescriptions, and increased hospitalizations, as laid out in one analysis of American Community Survey data.[38]

This instability not only affects renters but homeowners as well. Data from the 2006 and 2008 Health and Retirement Study, which captured mortgage delinquency, showed that individuals with delinquent mortgage payments were more likely to have fair/poor self-rated health at baseline and more likely to experience cost-related decreased medication taking and a decline in health as measured by elevated depressive symptoms and decreased medication taking.[39]

Fortunately, there are numerous interventions at the local, state, and federal levels to address high housing costs. Examples include onetime rental assistance payments and housing voucher programs. The federal Housing Choice Voucher Program (commonly known as the Section 8 program) is one of the largest federal housing assistance programs and currently assists more than 2 million families. There are local and state variations on parameters for the vouchers, but broadly, the goal of the program is to pay all rent up to the point of 30% of household income.

There is evidence that housing vouchers may mitigate some of the health harms of housing affordability previously noted. Those receiving rental assistance experience significantly less psychological distress than those not receiving assistance,[40] and studies have shown that receiving rental assistance is associated with better self-rated health[41] and reduced days of school absence[42]; however, the relationship may be more complex and requires further examination.[43]

Despite the broad scope of these rental assistance programs, there are still many barriers to both obtaining and using housing vouchers. These barriers include the limited number of vouchers, landlords refusing to accept vouchers as payment, and ongoing high cost of rent, despite assistance.[44] They mean that thousands of families across the country still deal with the burden of high housing costs despite these programs.

Finally, while there is evidence of the financial trade-offs that families may make because of the high cost of housing, there is less empirical data on the myriad of other trade-offs that families may make because of housing costs. These include living farther away from work or school to cut costs or disrupting social networks to make housing decisions based on cost. Further exploration of the mental and health impacts of stress from rent burden is also required.

Key Concept

Even for families that can stay housed, the high cost of housing can contribute to worse health outcomes, primarily by reducing the availability of financial resources for other health-related needs.

Clinicians can support patients facing housing affordability issues by

- **Connecting patients to local rental assistance programs**
- **Assessing cost burden when exploring issues such as medication taking practices or missed appointments**
- **Supporting local legislation and advocacy efforts to regulate housing costs**

Housing Stability/Insecurity

Mounting housing costs and untenable, unsafe conditions make it increasingly difficult for low-income and marginalized people to stay stably housed. Although there is not a commonly recognized definition of housing stability, it is broadly conceived of as the cluster of interconnected factors affecting a person's ability to choose to remain where they are living or to choose to leave of their own volition. These factors include issues of cost and housing conditions, as noted in the Housing Quality/Conditions and Housing Affordability/Cost sections earlier in this chapter and are most acutely represented by forced relocations such as

- **Eviction:** Forced removal of person for place of residence initiated by landlord.
- **Foreclosure:** Forced relocation of a homeowner when a bank or lending agency repossesses a property.

Researchers at the Princeton Eviction Lab have begun to centralize eviction data to show national eviction patterns. In 2018, their analysis showed that an estimated 3.6 million eviction cases were filed. Their data also allow them to look for regional variations. The region with the highest eviction rates (number of household evictions per 100 residential households) in 2016 was North Charleston, SC, at 16.5%, meaning that in North Charleston, in 2016, 16.5 of every 100 households faced eviction.

There are disparities in who is affected by evictions. Eviction rates were higher among Black and Hispanic neighborhoods, even when controlling for poverty and segregation. Female heads of a household were also more likely to be evicted in Black neighborhoods but not in white or Hispanic neighborhoods.[45]

There are substantial data showing the immense impact that eviction can have on a family.[45–47] Eviction forces a family out of its home, and in the process of eviction, families often lose possessions, including documents and medications. There is also a growing body of literature revealing that forced moves and evictions directly affect physical and mental health. Specifically, existing data show negative impacts of eviction on birthing parent and child health, including higher rates of birthing parent depression, lower gestational ages, lower birth weights, and a trend toward increased infant mortality.[48,49] The data also suggested that material hardship and birthing parent depression persisted as much as 2 years[46] after the completed eviction. Although the impact of eviction on specific health conditions needs to be further explored, there is evidence of eviction affecting chronic disease management and infection transmission, specifically associations with poorer HIV viral load management[50] and increased risk for sexually transmitted infection transmission.[51]

The impacts are also strongly felt among homeowners who experience foreclosure. The economic recession of 2008 saw a spike in foreclosures, the impact of which has only recently begun to be explored. Data on foreclosures between 2005 and 2009 show a disproportionate impact on Black and Latine households and possibly even a contribution to racial residential segregation.[52] An American Heart Association study showed that Latine people in residential areas at higher risk for foreclosure experience higher rates of hypertension and hyperlipidemia than those in areas with lower foreclosure risk[53] (**Box 6-5**).

A direct result and corollary of housing instability is the state of homelessness. The health impacts of homelessness are well-documented, including both the exacerbation of common acute and chronic disease that is worsened by homelessness and the specific conditions that are uniquely threatening to people experiencing chronic homelessness. A multicenter study of people

Box 6-5.
Housing and Health in the Era of COVID-19

The COVID-19 pandemic highlighted the way in which a person's access to safe, stable housing can affect their health.

One marked finding through the early data of the pandemic was the disparities in SARS-CoV-2 transmission and mortality across different racial groups. Reflecting historical segregationist practices, analyses have shown an association between historically redlined neighborhoods with higher risk for COVID-19.[a]

Not only was vulnerability to COVID-19 correlated with existing patterns of housing inequality, but interventions to address housing risk were correlated with decreased rates of COVID-19 incidence and mortality. Through the early years of the pandemic, many states instituted a moratorium on evictions, meaning that eviction cases did not move forward for a set period. Studies that explored this intervention showed that states lifting their eviction bans earlier faced higher rates of COVID-19 incidence and mortality[b] than those maintaining their eviction moratorium.

Finally, the COVID-19 pandemic had a particular impact on people experiencing homelessness. The increased risk for infection in people experiencing homelessness is multifactorial; in addition to the high rates of preexisting chronic disease, the setting of congregate shelter and the lack of stable quarantine options have made people experiencing homelessness particularly vulnerable to SARS-CoV-2 transmission and infection. Recent epidemiological studies revealed significantly increased mortality rates among people experiencing homelessness.[c]

[a] Li M, Yuan F. Historical redlining and resident exposure to COVID-19: a study of New York City. *Race Soc Probl.* 2022;14(2):85–100.

[b] Leifheit KM, Linton SL, Raifman J, et al. Expiring eviction moratoriums and COVID-19 incidence and mortality. *Am J Epidemiol.* 2021;190(12):2503–2510.

[c] Porter NAC, Brosnan HK, Chang AH, Henwood BF, Kuhn R. Race and ethnicity and sex variation in COVID-19 mortality risks among adults experiencing homelessness in Los Angeles County, California. *JAMA Netw Open.* 2022;5(12):e2245263.

experiencing homelessness in Canada shows that mortality is higher among people experiencing homelessness, although the specific reason why remains unclear. Likely, it is a result of the myriad health harms faced by people experiencing homelessness.[54] Other conditions with specific risks for people experiencing homelessness include exposure injuries, from specific environmental harms and from extreme weather, as well as foot injuries and wounds.[55] The American Academy of Pediatrics (AAP) policy statement on homelessness identifies several of the physical and mental health harms faced by children experiencing homelessness. It also makes a number of recommendations regarding care for such children, such as developing tools to identify homelessness and housing insecurity among patients and optimizing acute care visits when possible to provide comprehensive care for patients with limited access to care.[56]

Key Concept

Housing instability, most notably forced evictions and foreclosures, has severe consequences for mental and physical health.

Clinicians can support patients facing housing instability by

- **Familiarizing themselves with local tenants' rights to ensure that patients and families facing eviction are aware of their rights and resources**
- **Providing medical documentation to support patients and families in housing court**
- **Participating in medical-legal partnerships (MLPs) that link patients and families to legal resources**
- **Supporting local legislation that addresses wrongful evictions and tenant protections (eg, Right to Counsel legislation)**

Neighborhood Effects

Because of the systemic discrimination and exclusion discussed in the Racism and Housing section earlier in this chapter, communities across the United States are segregated in their residential patterns. Decades of disinvestment and differential resource allocation has meant that the neighborhoods that are primarily Black and Latine are more likely to experience poverty and to have fewer health-related resources, such as access to stores with healthy food, spaces for recreation, and access to quality education, and are more likely to face health harms such as freeways and environmental hazards.[57,58]

Many of these exposures can be broadly categorized as features of the built environment, such as buildings, parks, roads, and other elements of community design that make up a neighborhood. These elements affect health in myriad ways. Transportation infrastructure affects road safety, walkability, and physical activity,[59] as well as access to health care services; availability of green spaces is associated with improved mental health scores,[60] and availability of affordable food options is linked to dietary habits and obesity.[61] Furthermore, in the current climate crisis, conscientious community design plays a key role in fortifying communities against weather and climate-related hazards. The built environment is increasingly being recognized as a core determinant of health, as noted in a January 2024 policy statement from the AAP. This policy statement provides a number of recommendations for health care providers to account for the health effects of the built environment and to advocate for design practices and institutional strategies that support health-promoting environments.[62] Given that a person's housing options are intrinsically connected to the built environment around them, these environmental and neighborhood factors can be considered part of the health impact of housing.

How the built environment and other features of a person's neighborhood affect health is complex, involving the material resources available in said neighborhood, mobility within and between neighborhoods, and the role of social relationships within neighborhoods and communities. Conceptual frameworks to explain these dynamics largely involve the feedback between the material resources, the physical and social environments of a neighborhood, and the way they influence health-related behaviors as well as ongoing stress and "weathering," the repeated exposure to social and economic adversity and political marginalization, itself affecting health (**Figure 6-4**).[63,64] There are also numerous methodological concerns regarding how these neighborhood effects are understood and measured. One way of reconciling these issues that has been proposed is to conceptualize neighborhood effects as *environmental exposure* effects,[64] as one might conceptualize physical exposures that affect health.

Keeping this idea of environmental exposure in mind, researchers have used tools such as spatial mapping to directly measure physical and social features of a neighborhood and then relate these exposures to health. In this context, there are numerous observational studies linking specific health outcomes to physical and social environmental features. These features can be subdivided into specific domains explored by the literature. Some examples are discussed in **Box 6-6**.

In addition to conducting observational studies, researchers have attempted to define a causal relationship between neighborhood characteristics and health via experimental conditions or natural experiments that involve movement from one neighborhood environment to another. One of the most well-known studies among these is the Moving to Opportunity for Fair Housing study, a multisite randomized controlled trial of the impact of residential mobility on various health and socioeconomic outcomes. Families in the experimental group of the study received a housing voucher to move to a low-poverty neighborhood, while families in the control group received traditional Section 8 housing vouchers or remained on the voucher waiting list.[65] Movement to low-poverty

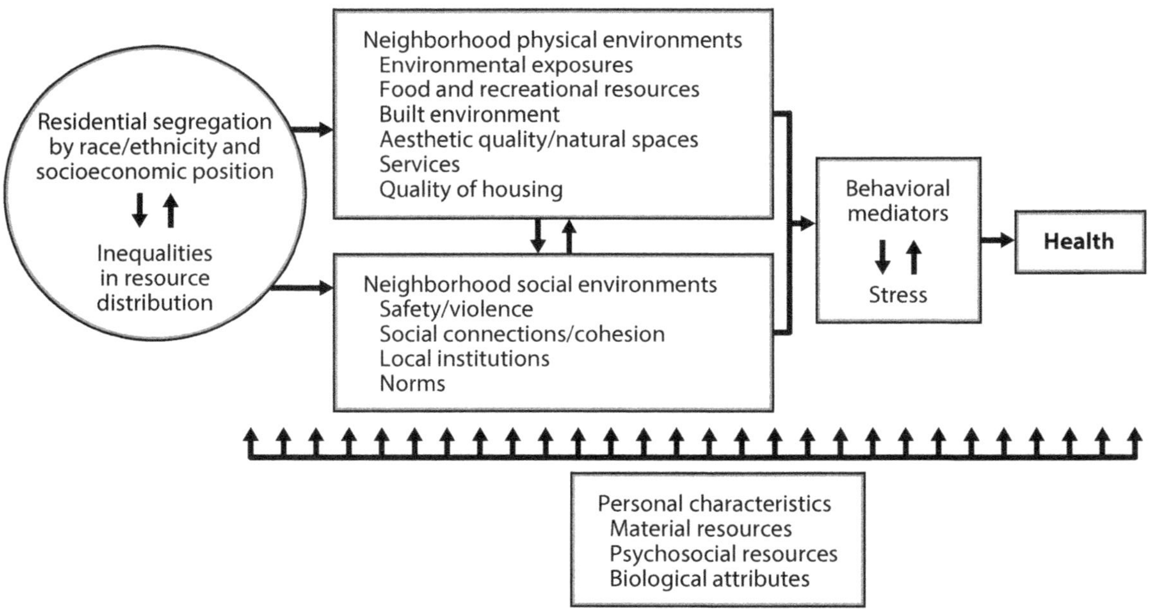

Figure 6-4. Conceptual Schema for Effects of Neighborhood on Health

From Diez Roux AV, Mair C. Neighborhood and health. *Ann N Y Acad Sci*. 2010;1186(1):125–145. Reprinted by permission of John Wiley and Sons.

neighborhoods was associated with lower hemoglobin A_{1c} level and lower body mass index[66] but had no effects on chronic disease measures[67] and variable effects on psychological health.[65,68] A 2016 analysis of the Moving to Opportunity study showed that children who moved to lower-poverty neighborhoods had greater economic earnings as adults than those who remained in higher-poverty neighborhoods, highlighting the long-term social impacts of these neighborhood effects.[69]

Box 6-6.
Examples of Domains of Neighborhoods Effects

Physical activity: A review of 50 studies showed that the presence of physical recreation resources is associated with physical activity in neighborhoods.[a]

Diet/food access: A rapidly growing body of literature is connecting density of food resources, specifically supermarkets, to healthier diets.[b]

Mental health: Depression is the most common outcome evaluated and has been associated with various markers of physical disorder in a neighborhood or neighborhood disturbances (eg, traffic, noise).

Cardiovascular health: Various neighborhood effects (eg, food resources, physical recreation resources, perceptions of safety and social cohesion) have all been found, in large epidemiological studies, to be associated with global cardiovascular health scores.

[a] Kaczynski AT, Henderson KA. Parks and recreation settings and active living: a review of associations with physical activity function and intensity. *J Phys Act Health.* 2008;5(4):619–632.

[b] Caspi CE, Sorensen G, Subramanian SV, Kawachi I. The local food environment and diet: a systematic review. *Health Place.* 2012;18(5):1172–1187.

Key Concept

Numerous observational studies make clear that features of the built and social environment are associated with a diverse array of health outcomes. Given the degree of segregation between neighborhoods, these associations suggest that neighborhood effects play a role in ongoing disparities in health outcomes.

Clinicians can address the neighborhood effects of housing with their patients by

- **Familiarizing themselves with local resources in the communities in which they practice**
- **Understanding how housing-related needs may suggest the presence of other health-related social needs (HRSNs)**
- **Advocating in partnership with community members who promote health and wellness for health-promoting design practices such as high-quality green space and recreational areas, open and safe bike lanes, and mixed-use development**
- **Advocating within their own institutions about strategies to increase sustainable and inclusive community development**

Screening for Housing Issues in Clinical Settings

Given the association between housing and physical and mental health, it has become a growing priority in health systems to identify patients with unstable or unsafe housing. Because of its recognized importance on health outcomes, housing is frequently identified as a core HRSN in a number of validated screening tools.[70–72] The AAP policy statement on poverty and child health recommends screening for risk factors within social determinants of health during clinical encounters, including housing.[73] The most common measures of housing in social needs screening tools are measures of housing quality, housing insecurity/instability, or some combination of the two. Measures of instability are used to capture the broad range of experiences that fall under the housing stability/insecurity mechanism discussed earlier in this chapter. Usually, they involve some variation of whether a patient can stay where they reside within a specified time frame, if they are currently living or recently lived in a shelter or on the street, or, simply, in the patient's own judgment, if they are in stable housing. Some measures of quality ask about perceptions of quality, while others ask about specific housing quality risks (eg, pests, cleanliness, lighting, mold, utilities, heating). The Centers for Medicare & Medicaid Services Accountable Health Communities Health-Related Social Needs Screening Tool assesses social needs across 5 main domains and includes 2 questions assessing living situation.[74] It asks participants to assess their ability to stay in their current living situation and asks them to identify the presence of specific risks, such as pests, mold, or heating and appliance issues. It should be noted that discordance between different housing measures has been described,[75] so when choosing a screening tool, clinicians should consider which elements of housing risk are of particular interest or what resources for intervention might exist. In whatever form, housing instability and quality are often frequently identified as among the most common needs.[71,76,77] Furthermore, housing needs identified through these screening tools have been associated with poor health outcomes and presence of other social needs across various clinical settings.[78,79]

In addition to tools to screen for social needs in the general population, there are efforts to create specific screening tools for housing needs, specifically to identify those most at risk for homelessness. For example, the Veterans Affairs (VA) health system has made a concerted effort to identify the risk for homelessness in its patient population. In 2012, the VA implemented a universal screening for homelessness in the electronic health record (EHR) in all its outpatient clinics (**Box 6-7**). This involved a system-wide, EHR-based prompt to screen all patients in the outpatient setting. The first year of this screening implementation showed that among respondents who were not already part of the homeless service system, recent prevalence of homelessness was at 0.9% and risk of homelessness was at 1.2%.[80] Similar tools have been developed for the ED, as the ED is often a setting in which individuals experiencing homelessness interact with the medical system. A 2-item screening tool for homelessness assessing self-perceived risk for future instability was found to be predictive of future shelter entry (**Box 6-7**).[81] Of note, qualitative evaluation with patients has shown general acceptance of this screening in the ED setting and may have other benefits beyond addressing unmet social needs, including supporting therapeutic rapport.[82] These examples demonstrate evidence for potential benefits of screening for housing insecurity in adult at-risk populations. Similarly, screening tools have been developed for use in the pediatric clinical setting. The IHELP pediatric social history tool (https://sirenetwork.ucsf.edu/tools-resources/resources/ihelp-pediatric-social-history-tool) can be used to screen families on their risk for housing insecurity via questions such as "Do you have concerns about being evicted or not being able to pay the rent?" and "Do you have concerns about not being

Box 6-7.
Examples of Housing Needs Screening Tools

Veterans Affairs Homelessness Screening Clinical Reminder[a]

- In the past 2 months, have you been living in stable housing that you own, rent, or stay in as part of a household? (A negative response indicates housing instability.)
- Are you worried or concerned that in the next 2 months you may not have stable housing that you own, rent, or stay in as part of a household? (A positive response indicates risk.)

Example Housing Risk Screening Tool for Emergency Department Use[b]

- Are you worried or concerned that in the next 2 months you may not have stable housing that you own, rent, or stay in as part of a household? (yes/no)
- How likely do you think it would be that you would have to use a homeless shelter in the next 6 months? (very unlikely to very likely)

[a] Montgomery AE, Fargo JD, Byrne TH, Kane VR, Culhane DP. Universal screening for homelessness and risk for homelessness in the Veterans Health Administration. *Am J Public Health*. 2013;103(suppl 2):S210–S211.

[b] Byrne T, Hoang M, Montgomery AE, et al. Performance of 2 single-item screening questions to identify future homelessness among emergency department patients. *JAMA Netw Open*. 2022;5(8):e2226691.

able to pay your mortgage?" The Health Leads Screening Toolkit also includes a housing security question ("Are you worried that in the next 2 months you may not have stable housing?") in its screening questionnaire. (Refer to **Figure 4-1**.)

Given the high prevalence of housing needs, especially in specific clinical settings, and the likely benefit of identifying these needs in clinical settings, it is perhaps worth considering why screening for housing needs is *not* more widespread. Indeed, a review of social needs screening and intervention tools in the ED setting showed that only 3% of reviewed literature specifically addressed housing needs.[83] Although there is limited research on specific barriers to implementing screening for housing needs in the clinical setting, it is likely they align with barriers for social needs screening in general, particularly limited resources and time to enact screening, challenging coordination with existing workflows, and lack of confidence in ability to address a positive screening result.[84] This lack of confidence in ability to address a need is likely heightened in the context of housing needs, given the labyrinthine process for navigating housing services in most states and the scarcity of affordable housing discussed in the Housing Stock section earlier in this chapter. When implementation of social needs screening tools is successful, flexible integration into workflow to align with local needs and resources, the presence of a specific social needs advocate, and external incentives such as targeting funding have been found to be facilitating factors.[85] As the VA example shows, integration of a simple, focused screening tool is possible and has potential for significant social and clinical impact; retrospective review from a VA sample shows that use of homelessness prevention services was associated with reduced all-cause mortality.[80] Identifying strategies to implement such screening into regular clinical practice should thus be considered a priority.

Key Concept

There are numerous validated tools for identifying housing needs in clinical settings. These primarily focus on housing quality and housing stability. When these tools are used, they often identify high rates of housing concerns. Targeted screening for housing instability for specific patient populations or in specific settings may be another route for identifying patient populations particularly at risk for housing needs.

Addressing Housing Needs in Clinical Settings

With the evidence of the role of housing in health outcomes, and the ability to identify these needs in clinical settings, there are growing efforts to develop interventions to meet housing needs in the clinical environment (**Figure 6-5**). Some of these interventions involve linking patients to existing community-based resources, while others attempt to provide comprehensive resources within the clinic setting itself.

Interventions focused on resource referral vary broadly in scope and intensity, from providing paper handouts and resource lists during the span of the provider visit to longitudinal patient navigation with social workers or CHWs.[70,71,86] There are growing attempts to evaluate the impact of these interventions, on both housing- and health-related outcomes; however, challenges include the degree of heterogeneity in these interventions, and thus far, there has been more focus on process outcomes than distal health outcomes.[87,88] Some data show a positive impact

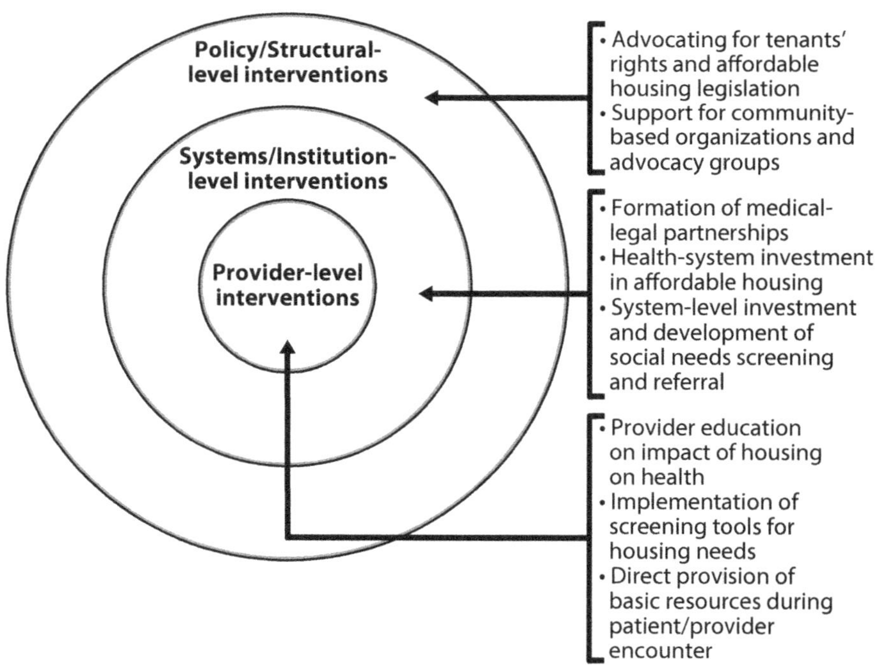

Figure 6-5. How Health Care Professionals and Systems Can Work to Address Unmet Housing Needs at Various Levels of Intervention

of these interventions on distal outcomes. One study in a pediatric practice shows that using a clinic-based resource referral program leads to reduced shelter placement for families,[71] and when surveyed, most patients in one large health system supported the use of social needs screening and their role in health outcomes.[89] As with screening for social needs, implementation of such resource delivery interventions requires dedicated time and resources. In some health systems, the use of CHWs as dedicated staff to address social needs has shown promise[76,90] and alleviates the need for the clinician to fit these discussions into the clinical encounter. At the same time, experience from existing interventions shows the need for clinical champions or advocates to highlight the importance of social needs interventions in the clinical setting and to shift practice culture to center social care as part of clinical care.[91]

Another form of intervention with a growing evidence base is MLPs. This model involves direct collaboration between clinical providers and legal providers, providing training to allow clinicians to see the legal implications and antecedents of clinical problems and allowing for direct connection to legal assistance and intervention to address a patient's social environment. Both qualitative and quantitative evidence suggest that the use of MLPs provides unique opportunities to identify and address the root social causes of clinical concerns, to make explicit the connections between a patient's health and legal and social environments, and, ultimately, to improve rates of connection to housing-related resources and, in one study, mental health outcomes as well.[92,93] Although there are, of course, hurdles to developing such a partnership from scratch, there are also a number tools to facilitate new MLPs. The National Center for Medical-Legal Partnership with the Milken Institute School of Public Health at the George Washington University has numerous resources, including a step-by-step toolkit on forming new partnerships, to help support clinicians and health care systems in developing their own partnership.[94]

The resource landscape available to patients and clinicians is shaped by local, state, and federal housing policy decisions. As such, physicians may also play a role in addressing the housing needs of patients by supporting legislative advocacy efforts to expand access to safe, affordable housing, using their voice to identify the link between housing needs and health outcomes. Through a combination of direct resource provision, interdisciplinary and interprofessional partnerships, and focused advocacy, health care professionals and systems may be able to support patients in addressing ongoing unmet housing needs.

Key Concept

There are efforts to develop interventions on housing needs in the clinical setting; however, ongoing evaluation of the impact of clinic-based housing interventions is still needed.

Medical-legal partnerships offer one example of cross-discipline and interprofessional collaboration that may serve as an effective model for addressing social needs in the clinical setting.

Engaging in political or legislative advocacy to highlight the health impacts of affordable housing policy is another role physicians can play in expanding access to housing resources for patients.

Conclusions and Recommendations

Safe, affordable, stable housing is a key component of multiple facets of individual and community lives—as a foundation for wealth generation, a space for social gathering, and, as is increasingly evident, a foundation of physical and mental health. Unfortunately, decades of discriminatory policy and practice, increasing housing costs, and lack of availability of safe housing stock have meant that it is increasingly difficult for people to maintain safe, stable housing, particularly those in marginalized communities.

Based on the existing evidence, core ways that clinicians can support patients with housing issues fall into 3 main domains. Within the patient encounter level, providers should recognize the prevalence of housing stability and quality issues among patients, particularly patients from historically marginalized communities. Implementing universal screening for housing issues by using validated tools can help identify these concerns and is the first step to addressing these social determinants of health. For patients with unmanaged chronic disease, poor medication taking, and persistent mental health concerns, broadening the differential diagnosis to include social barriers can further help address these upstream causes of poor health.

At the institutional and community levels, providers can familiarize themselves with local community-based resources and social service infrastructure to identify resources patients can connect to. As the need for screening for social needs and referral for services is being increasingly recognized, health systems are developing systems to increase resource linkage in clinical practice. Providers can work within their institutions to develop and implement such screening and referral systems, with a focus on identifying housing-related issues and resources.

At the advocacy level, as previously described, the root causes of our current housing crisis are related to local and federal policy decisions. Across the country, there are ongoing efforts among communities, advocates, and policymakers to rethink our housing system in a way that ensures safe, affordable, stable housing for all. Given the association between housing and health as described in this chapter, health care professionals can play an important role in highlighting the impacts of poor housing and can support advocacy efforts in their local communities to ensure that they prioritize the needs of our patients most vulnerable to the health harms of social inequity.

Key Points

- Housing is currently at a crisis in the United States, particularly for patients in families with low incomes and patients in marginalized communities.
- Our current housing crisis has its roots in histories of racially discriminatory practices and long-term disinvestment in public strategies for affordable housing.
- Housing is related to mental and physical health outcomes along a number of different pathways, specifically housing quality/conditions, housing affordability/cost, housing stability/insecurity, and neighborhood effects.
- Screening for housing needs in the health care setting can help identify risk factors for poor health outcomes.
- Multidisciplinary solutions such as medical-legal clinics and embedded CHWs are promising avenues through which health care professionals and health systems can work to address housing needs in clinical settings.

References

1. Joint Center for Housing Studies. *America's Rental Housing 2022*. Harvard University; 2022
2. *The GAP: A Shortage of Affordable Homes*. National Low Income Housing Coalition; 2022. Accessed May 3, 2024. https://nlihc.org/gap
3. Rothstein R. *The Color of Law: A Forgotten History of How Our Government Segregated America*. Liveright Publishing Corp; 2017
4. Rothstein R. Race and public housing: revisiting the federal role. Economic Policy Institute. December 17, 2012. Accessed May 3, 2024. https://www.epi.org/publication/race-public-housing-revisiting-federal-role
5. Gerken M, Batko S, Fallon K, Fernandez E, Williams A, Chen B. *Assessing the Legacies of Historical Redlining: Correlations with Measures of Modern Housing Instability*. Urban Institute; 2023
6. De Los Santos H, Jiang K, Bernardi J, Okechukwu C. From redlining to gentrification: the policy of the past that affects health outcomes today. Harvard Medical School Center for Primary Care. May 26, 2021. Accessed May 3, 2024. https://info.primarycare.hms.harvard.edu/review/redlining-gentrification-health-outcomes
7. Li M, Yuan F. Historical redlining and resident exposure to COVID-19: a study of New York City. *Race Soc Probl*. 2022;14(2):85–100 PMID: 34178163 doi: 10.1007/s12552-021-09338-z
8. Welsh NH. Racially restrictive covenants in the United States: a call to action. *Agora J Urban Plan Des*. 2018:130–142
9. Rothwell JT, Massey DS. Density zoning and class segregation in U.S. metropolitan areas. *Soc Sci Q*. 2010;91(5):1123–1143 PMID: 21117332 doi: 10.1111/j.1540-6237.2010.00724.x
10. Rothwell J, Massey DS. The effect of density zoning on racial segregation in U.S. urban areas. *Urban Aff Rev*. 2009;44(6):779–806 PMID: 25009413 doi: 10.1177/1078087409334163
11. Rouse C, Bernstein J, Knudsen H, Zhang J. Exclusionary zoning: its effect on racial discrimination in the housing market. *White House Council of Economic Advisers* blog. June 17, 2021. Accessed May 3, 2024. https://www.whitehouse.gov/cea/written-materials/2021/06/17/exclusionary-zoning-its-effect-on-racial-discrimination-in-the-housing-market
12. Kazis N. *Ending Exclusionary Zoning in New York City's Suburbs*. NYU Furman Center; 2020. Accessed May 3, 2024. https://furmancenter.org/files/Ending_Exclusionary_Zoning_in_New_York_Citys_Suburbs.pdf
13. HUD history. US Department of Housing and Urban Development. Accessed May 3, 2024. https://www.hud.gov/about/hud_history
14. Shashaty AS. U.S. cuts back and shifts course on housing aid. *New York Times*. October 18, 1981. Accessed May 3, 2024. https://www.nytimes.com/1981/10/18/realestate/us-cuts-back-and-shifts-course-on-housing-aid.html
15. Public housing history. National Low Income Housing Coalition. October 17, 2019. Accessed May 3, 2024. https://nlihc.org/resource/public-housing-history
16. Investors buy record share of homes in 2021, increasing rental prices. National Low Income Housing Coalition. February 28, 2022. Accessed May 3, 2024. https://nlihc.org/resource/investors-buy-record-share-homes-2021-increasing-rental-prices
17. Vogell H. When private equity becomes your landlord. ProPublica. February 7, 2022. Accessed May 3, 2024. https://www.propublica.org/article/when-private-equity-becomes-your-landlord
18. Farrell M. Blackstone expands further into rental housing in the United States. *New York Times*. February 16, 2022. Accessed May 3, 2024. https://www.nytimes.com/2022/02/16/business/blackstone-real-estate-acquisition.html
19. Homes Guarantee. Accessed May 3, 2024. https://homesguarantee.com
20. Taylor L. Housing and health: an overview of the literature. *Health Aff Policy Brief*. June 7, 2018. Accessed October 17, 2024. https://www.healthaffairs.org/content/briefs/housing-and-health-overview-literature

21. Hu M, Zhang K, Nguyen QC, Tasdizen T, Krusche KU. A multistate study on housing factors influential to heat-related illness in the United States. *Int J Environ Res Public Health*. 2022;19(23):15762 PMID: 36497839 doi: 10.3390/ijerph192315762

22. Yeter D, Banks EC, Aschner M. Disparity in risk factor severity for early childhood blood lead among predominantly African-American Black children: the 1999 to 2010 US NHANES. *Int J Environ Res Public Health*. 2020;17(5):1552 PMID: 32121216 doi: 10.3390/ijerph17051552

23. Teye SO, Yanosky JD, Cuffee Y, et al. Exploring persistent racial/ethnic disparities in lead exposure among American children aged 1–5 years: results from NHANES 1999–2016. *Int Arch Occup Environ Health*. 2021;94(4):723–730 PMID: 33394180 doi: 10.1007/s00420-020-01616-4

24. Hauptman M, Rogers ML, Scarpaci M, Morin B, Vivier PM. Neighborhood disparities and the burden of lead poisoning. *Pediatr Res*. 2023;94(2):826–836 PMID: 36899126 doi: 10.1038/s41390-023-02476-7

25. Lanphear BP, Kahn RS, Berger O, Auinger P, Bortnick SM, Nahhas RW. Contribution of residential exposures to asthma in US children and adolescents. *Pediatrics*. 2001;107(6):e98 PMID: 11389296 doi: 10.1542/peds.107.6.e98

26. Rauh VA, Landrigan PJ, Claudio L. Housing and health: intersection of poverty and environmental exposures. *Ann N Y Acad Sci*. 2008;1136(1):276–288 PMID: 18579887 doi: 10.1196/annals.1425.032

27. Pacheco CM, Ciaccio CE, Nazir N, et al. Homes of low-income minority families with asthmatic children have increased condition issues. *Allergy Asthma Proc*. 2014;35(6):467–474 PMID: 25584914 doi: 10.2500/aap.2014.35.3792

28. Lemire E, Samuels EA, Wang W, Haber A. Unequal housing conditions and code enforcement contribute to asthma disparities in Boston, Massachusetts. *Health Aff (Millwood)*. 2022;41(4):563–572 PMID: 35377754 doi: 10.1377/hlthaff.2021.01403

29. Runyan CW, Casteel C, Perkis D, et al. Unintentional injuries in the home in the United States, I: mortality. *Am J Prev Med*. 2005;28(1):73–79 PMID: 15626560 doi: 10.1016/j.amepre.2004.09.010

30. Cardoza JE, Gronlund CJ, Schott J, Ziegler T, Stone B, O'Neill MS. Heat-related illness is associated with lack of air conditioning and pre-existing health problems in Detroit, Michigan, USA: a community-based participatory co-analysis of survey data. *Int J Environ Res Public Health*. 2020;17(16):5704 PMID: 32784593 doi: 10.3390/ijerph17165704

31. Evans J, Hyndman S, Stewart-Brown S, Smith D, Petersen S. An epidemiological study of the relative importance of damp housing in relation to adult health. *J Epidemiol Community Health*. 2000;54(9):677–686 PMID: 10942447 doi: 10.1136/jech.54.9.677

32. Howden-Chapman P, Crane J, Matheson A, et al. Retrofitting houses with insulation to reduce health inequalities: aims and methods of a clustered, randomised community-based trial. *Soc Sci Med*. 2005;61(12):2600–2610 PMID: 16061320 doi: 10.1016/j.socscimed.2005.04.049

33. Thomson H, Thomas S, Sellstrom E, Petticrew M. Housing improvements for health and associated socio-economic outcomes. *Cochrane Database Syst Rev*. 2013;(2):CD008657 PMID: 23450585 doi: 10.1002/14651858.CD008657.pub2

34. Drehobl A, Ross L, Ayala R. *How High Are Household Energy Burdens?* American Council for an Energy-Efficient Economy; 2020. Accessed May 3, 2024. https://www.aceee.org/research-report/u2006

35. Frank DA, Neault NB, Skalicky A, et al. Heat or eat: the Low Income Home Energy Assistance Program and nutritional and health risks among children less than 3 years of age. *Pediatrics*. 2006;118(5):e1293–e1302 PMID: 17079530 doi: 10.1542/peds.2005-2943

36. Pollack CE, Griffin BA, Lynch J. Housing affordability and health among homeowners and renters. *Am J Prev Med*. 2010;39(6):515–521 PMID: 21084071 doi: 10.1016/j.amepre.2010.08.002

37. Meltzer R, Schwartz A. Housing affordability and health: evidence from New York City. *Hous Policy Debate*. 2016;26(1):80–104 doi: 10.1080/10511482.2015.1020321

38. Kushel MB, Gupta R, Gee L, Haas JS. Housing instability and food insecurity as barriers to health care among low-income Americans. *J Gen Intern Med.* 2006;21(1):71–77 PMID: 16423128 doi: 10.1111/j.1525-1497.2005.00278.x

39. Alley DE, Lloyd J, Pagán JA, Pollack CE, Shardell M, Cannuscio C. Mortgage delinquency and changes in access to health resources and depressive symptoms in a nationally representative cohort of Americans older than 50 years. *Am J Public Health.* 2011;101(12):2293–2298 PMID: 22021301 doi: 10.2105/AJPH.2011.300245

40. Denary W, Fenelon A, Schlesinger P, Purtle J, Blankenship KM, Keene DE. Does rental assistance improve mental health? insights from a longitudinal cohort study. *Soc Sci Med.* 2021;282:114100 PMID: 34144434 doi: 10.1016/j.socscimed.2021.114100

41. Keene DE, Niccolai L, Rosenberg A, Schlesinger P, Blankenship KM. Rental assistance and adult self-rated health. *J Health Care Poor Underserved.* 2020;31(1):325–339 PMID: 32037334 doi: 10.1353/hpu.2020.0025

42. Fenelon A, Boudreaux M, Slopen N, Newman SJ. The benefits of rental assistance for children's health and school attendance in the United States. *Demography.* 2021;58(4):1171–1195 PMID: 33970240 doi: 10.1215/00703370-9305166

43. Antonakos CL, Colabianchi N. Impact of rental assistance on modifiable health risk factors and behaviors in adults. *Cityscape.* 2018;20(2):133–144 PMID: 30761186

44. Miles DRB, Samuels B, Pollack CE. Leveraging housing vouchers to address health disparities. *Am J Public Health.* 2017;107(2):238–240 PMID: 28075648 doi: 10.2105/AJPH.2016.303565

45. Desmond M. Eviction and the reproduction of urban poverty. *Am J Sociol.* 2012;118(1):88–133

46. Desmond M, Kimbro RT. Eviction's fallout: housing, hardship, and health. *Soc Forces.* 2015;94(1):295–324 doi: 10.1093/sf/sov044

47. Desmond M, Gershenson C, Kiviat B. Forced relocation and residential instability among urban renters. *Soc Serv Rev.* 2015;89(2):227–262 doi: 10.1086/681091

48. Himmelstein G, Desmond M. Association of eviction with adverse birth outcomes among women in Georgia, 2000 to 2016. *JAMA Pediatr.* 2021;175(5):494–500 PMID: 33646291 doi: 10.1001/jamapediatrics.2020.6550

49. Hazekamp C, Yousuf S, Day K, Daly MK, Sheehan K. Eviction and pediatric health outcomes in Chicago. *J Community Health.* 2020;45(5):891–899 PMID: 32189213 doi: 10.1007/s10900-020-00806-y

50. Kennedy MC, Kerr T, McNeil R, et al. Residential eviction and risk of detectable plasma HIV-1 RNA viral load among HIV-positive people who use drugs. *AIDS Behav.* 2017;21(3):678–687 PMID: 26906022 doi: 10.1007/s10461-016-1315-z

51. Niccolai LM, Blankenship KM, Keene DE. Eviction from renter-occupied households and rates of sexually transmitted infections: a county-level ecological analysis. *Sex Transm Dis.* 2019;46(1):63–68 PMID: 30148755 doi: 10.1097/OLQ.0000000000000904

52. Hall M, Crowder K, Spring A. Neighborhood foreclosures, racial/ethnic transitions, and residential segregation. *Am Sociol Rev.* 2015;80(3):526–549 PMID: 26120142 doi: 10.1177/0003122415581334

53. Sims M, Kershaw KN, Breathett K, et al; American Heart Association Council on Epidemiology and Prevention and Council on Quality of Care and Outcomes Research. Importance of housing and cardiovascular health and well-being: a scientific statement from the American Heart Association. *Circ Cardiovasc Qual Outcomes.* 2020;13(8):e000089 PMID: 32673512 doi: 10.1161/HCQ.0000000000000089

54. Hwang SW, Wilkins R, Tjepkema M, O'Campo PJ, Dunn JR. Mortality among residents of shelters, rooming houses, and hotels in Canada: 11 year follow-up study. *BMJ.* 2009;339:b4036 PMID: 19858533 doi: 10.1136/bmj.b4036

55. Koh HK, O'Connell JJ. Improving health care for homeless people. *JAMA.* 2016;316(24):2586–2587 PMID: 28027356 doi: 10.1001/jama.2016.18760

56. American Academy of Pediatrics Council on Community Pediatrics. Providing care for children and adolescents facing homelessness and housing insecurity. *Pediatrics.* 2013;131(6):1206–1210 PMID: 23713108 doi: 10.1542/peds.2013-0645

57. Turner MA, Greene S. Causes and consequences of separate and unequal neighborhoods. Urban Institute. Accessed May 3, 2024. https://www.urban.org/racial-equity-analytics-lab/structural-racism-explainer-collection/causes-and-consequences-separate-and-unequal-neighborhoods

58. Williams DR, Collins C. Racial residential segregation: a fundamental cause of racial disparities in health. *Public Health Rep.* 2001;116(5):404–416 PMID: 12042604 doi: 10.1016/S0033-3549(04)50068-7

59. Lubans DR, Boreham CA, Kelly P, Foster CE. The relationship between active travel to school and health-related fitness in children and adolescents: a systematic review. *Int J Behav Nutr Phys Act.* 2011;8(1):5 PMID: 21269514 doi: 10.1186/1479-5868-8-5

60. Markevych I, Tiesler CMT, Fuertes E, et al. Access to urban green spaces and behavioural problems in children: results from the GINIplus and LISAplus studies. *Environ Int.* 2014;71:29–35 PMID: 24953038 doi: 10.1016/j.envint.2014.06.002

61. Huang H. A spatial analysis of obesity: interaction of urban food environments and racial segregation in Chicago. *J Urban Health.* 2021;98(5):676–686 PMID: 34264475 doi: 10.1007/s11524-021-00553-y

62. Bole A, Bernstein A, White MJ, et al; American Academy of Pediatrics Council on Environmental Health and Climate Change and Section on Minority Health, Equity, and Inclusion. The built environment and pediatric health. *Pediatrics.* 2024;153(1):e2023064772 PMID: 38105695 doi: 10.1542/peds.2023-064772

63. Ellen IG, Mijanovich T, Dillman KN. Neighborhood effects on health: exploring the links and assessing the evidence. *J Urban Aff.* 2001;23(3–4):391–408 doi: 10.1111/0735-2166.00096

64. Diez Roux AV, Mair C. Neighborhoods and health. *Ann N Y Acad Sci.* 2010;1186(1):125–145 PMID: 20201871 doi: 10.1111/j.1749-6632.2009.05333.x

65. Orr L, Feins JD, Jacob R, et al. *Moving to Opportunity for Fair Housing Demonstration Program: Interim Impacts Evaluation.* US Dept of Housing and Urban Development; 2003. Accessed September 27, 2024. https://www.huduser.gov/publications/pdf/mtofullreport.pdf

66. Ludwig J, Sanbonmatsu L, Gennetian L, et al. Neighborhoods, obesity, and diabetes—a randomized social experiment. *N Engl J Med.* 2011;365(16):1509–1519 PMID: 22010917 doi: 10.1056/NEJMsa1103216

67. Sanbonmatsu L, Ludwig J, Katz L, et al. *Moving to Opportunity for Fair Housing Demonstration Program: Final Impacts Evaluation.* US Dept of Housing and Urban Development; 2011. Accessed May 3, 2024. https://www.huduser.gov/publications/pdf/MTOFHD_fullreport_v2.pdf

68. Osypuk TL, Tchetgen EJ, Acevedo-Garcia D, et al. Differential mental health effects of neighborhood relocation among youth in vulnerable families: results from a randomized trial. *Arch Gen Psychiatry.* 2012;69(12):1284–1294 PMID: 23045214 doi: 10.1001/archgenpsychiatry.2012.449

69. Chetty R, Hendren N, Katz LF. The effects of exposure to better neighborhoods on children: new evidence from the Moving to Opportunity experiment. *Am Econ Rev.* 2016;106(4):855–902 PMID: 29546974 doi: 10.1257/aer.20150572

70. De La Vega PB, Losi S, Martinez LS, et al. Implementing THRIVE, an EHR-based screening and referral system to address social determinants of health (SDOH) in an urban safety net hospital. *J Gen Intern Med.* 2019;34(suppl 2):S736–S737 PMID: 31090026 doi: 10.1007/s11606-019-05007-5

71. Garg A, Toy S, Tripodis Y, Silverstein M, Freeman E. Addressing social determinants of health at well child care visits: a cluster RCT. *Pediatrics.* 2015;135(2):e296–e304 PMID: 25560448 doi: 10.1542/peds.2014-2888

72. Boch S, Keedy H, Chavez L, Dolce M, Chisolm D. An integrative review of social determinants of health screenings used in primary care settings. *J Health Care Poor Underserved.* 2020;31(2):603–622 PMID: 33410796 doi: 10.1353/hpu.2020.0048

73. American Academy of Pediatrics Council on Community Pediatrics. Poverty and child health in the United States. *Pediatrics.* 2016;137(4):e20160339 PMID: 26962238 doi: 10.1542/peds.2016-0339

74. Billioux A, Verlander K, Anthony S, Alley D. Standardized screening for health-related social needs in clinical settings: the Accountable Health Communities screening tool. *NAM Perspect.* 2017 doi: 10.31478/201705b

75. De Marchis EH, Ettinger de Cuba SA, Chang L, et al. Screening discordance and characteristics of patients with housing-related social risks. *Am J Prev Med.* 2021;61(1):e1–e12 PMID: 33785274 doi: 10.1016/j.amepre.2021.01.027

76. Fiori KP, Rehm CD, Sanderson D, et al. Integrating social needs screening and community health workers in primary care: the Community Linkage to Care program. *Clin Pediatr (Phila).* 2020;59(6):547–556 PMID: 32131620 doi: 10.1177/0009922820908589

77. Heller CG, Parsons AS, Chambers EC, Fiori KP, Rehm CD. Social risks among primary care patients in a large urban health system. *Am J Prev Med.* 2020;58(4):514–525 PMID: 32199514 doi: 10.1016/j.amepre.2019.11.011

78. Sandel M, Baeder A, Bradman A, et al. Housing interventions and control of health-related chemical agents: a review of the evidence. *J Public Health Manag Pract.* 2010;16(5)(suppl):S24–S33 PMID: 20689371 doi: 10.1097/PHH.0b013e3181e3cc2a

79. Wormley K, Dickson D, Alter H, Njoku N, Imani P, Anderson ES. Association of social needs and housing status among urban emergency department patients. *West J Emerg Med.* 2022;23(6):802–810 PMID: 36409947 doi: 10.5811/westjem.2022.8.55705

80. Montgomery AE, Fargo JD, Byrne TH, Kane VR, Culhane DP. Universal screening for homelessness and risk for homelessness in the Veterans Health Administration. *Am J Public Health.* 2013;103 (suppl 2):S210–S211 PMID: 24148032 doi: 10.2105/AJPH.2013.301398

81. Byrne T, Hoang M, Montgomery AE, et al. Performance of 2 single-item screening questions to identify future homelessness among emergency department patients. *JAMA Netw Open.* 2022;5(8):e2226691 PMID: 35969399 doi: 10.1001/jamanetworkopen.2022.26691

82. Kelly A, Fazio D, Padgett D, et al. Patient views on emergency department screening and interventions related to housing. *Acad Emerg Med.* 2022;29(5):589–597 PMID: 35064727 doi: 10.1111/acem.14442

83. Walter LA, Schoenfeld EM, Smith CH, et al. Emergency department–based interventions affecting social determinants of health in the United States: a scoping review. *Acad Emerg Med.* 2021;28(6):666–674 PMID: 33368833 doi: 10.1111/acem.14201

84. Schickedanz A, Hamity C, Rogers A, Sharp AL, Jackson A. Clinician experiences and attitudes regarding screening for social determinants of health in a large integrated health system. *Med Care.* 2019;57(6) (suppl 2):S197–S201 PMID: 31095061 doi: 10.1097/MLR.0000000000001051

85. Gruß I, Bunce A, Davis J, Dambrun K, Cottrell E, Gold R. Initiating and implementing social determinants of health data collection in community health centers. *Popul Health Manag.* 2021;24(1):52–58 PMID: 32119804 doi: 10.1089/pop.2019.0205

86. Manian N, Wagner CA, Placzek H, Darby BA, Kaiser TJ, Rog DJ. Relationship between intervention dosage and success of resource connections in a social needs intervention. *Public Health.* 2020;185:324–331 PMID: 32726729 doi: 10.1016/j.puhe.2020.05.058

87. Gottlieb LM, Wing H, Adler NE. A systematic review of interventions on patients' social and economic needs. *Am J Prev Med.* 2017;53(5):719–729 PMID: 28688725 doi: 10.1016/j.amepre.2017.05.011

88. Bickerdike L, Booth A, Wilson PM, Farley K, Wright K. Social prescribing: less rhetoric and more reality: a systematic review of the evidence. *BMJ Open.* 2017;7(4):e013384 PMID: 28389486 doi: 10.1136/bmjopen-2016-013384

89. Rogers AJ, Hamity C, Sharp AL, Jackson AH, Schickedanz AB. Patients' attitudes and perceptions regarding social needs screening and navigation: multi-site survey in a large integrated health system. *J Gen Intern Med.* 2020;35(5):1389–1395 PMID: 31898132 doi: 10.1007/s11606-019-05588-1

90. Rogers EA, Manser ST, Cleary J, Joseph AM, Harwood EM, Call KT. Integrating community health workers into medical homes. *Ann Fam Med.* 2018;16(1):14–20 PMID: 29311170 doi: 10.1370/afm.2171

91. Parulekar M, Rogers C. Identifying and addressing social determinants of health (SDOH) in ambulatory geriatric settings: workflow, results, challenges, and opportunities. *J Am Geriatr Soc*. 2020;68 (suppl 1):S44 doi: 10.1111/jgs.16431

92. Tsai J, Middleton M, Villegas J, et al. Medical-legal partnerships at Veterans Affairs medical centers improved housing and psychosocial outcomes for vets. *Health Aff (Millwood)*. 2017;36(12):2195–2203 PMID: 29200329 doi: 10.1377/hlthaff.2017.0759

93. Hernández D. "Extra oomph": addressing housing disparities through medical legal partnership interventions. *Housing Stud*. 2016;31(7):871–890 PMID: 27867247 doi: 10.1080/02673037.2016.1150431

94. Marple K, Curran M, Lawton E, Rahajason D. Bringing lawyers onto the health center care team to promote patient & community health. National Center for Medical-Legal Partnership. October 2020. Accessed May 3, 2024. https://medical-legalpartnership.org/wp-content/uploads/2020/10/Health-Center-MLP-Toolkit-FINAL.pdf

CHAPTER 7

Food Insecurity

Radhika Teli, MD; Michaela Domaratzky, MD; and Carol Duh-Leong, MD, MPP, FAAP

Food insecurity is defined as unstable and unreliable access to adequate, nutritious food. In the United States, at least 1 in 7 children experiences food insecurity. Because this critical social determinant of health can have negative implications on child health and development, it is important for pediatric practitioners to screen for, and identify, food insecurity in children and their households by using the Hunger Vital Sign. Food insecurity has been shown to disproportionately affect high-risk groups, including racially marginalized groups and homes headed by a single caregiver. In the clinical setting, food insecurity can present in various ways, including nutrition deficiencies, less optimal child feeding behaviors, poorer mental health and academic outcomes, and higher rates of emergency department use. This chapter also summarizes resources available at the local, state, and national levels to address food insecurity and outlines possible strategies for managing food insecurity in the clinic setting. As we expand our understanding of food insecurity in the pediatric population, recommendations on how to best approach it will continue to evolve.

CHAPTER 7

Food Insecurity

Radhika Teli, MD; Michaela Domaratzky, MD; and Carol Duh-Leong, MD, MPP, FAAP

Introduction

The term *food insecurity* refers to uncertain access to adequate, nutritious food, often because of limited financial resources. Studies show that 17.3% of US households with children and adolescents younger than 18 years, or 6.4 million children and adolescents, meet the US Department of Agriculture (USDA) definition of "food-insecure" in 2022.[1] The Food Research & Action Center (FRAC), a national organization that has been addressing food insecurity for decades, has highlighted that households with children younger than 6 years, headed by a single caregiver or coming from racially marginalized groups (eg, Black and Hispanic/Latino), are at particularly high risk of experiencing food insecurity.[2] Rates of food insecurity increased during the COVID-19 pandemic, likely exacerbating these disparities.[3] In 2020, 7.6% of households with children experienced food insecurity, an increase from 6.5% in 2019.[4]

Researchers have documented associations between food insecurity and negative child health outcomes. Pediatric practitioners are on the frontlines to recognize signs and symptoms of food insecurity, as well as to be able to mitigate food insecurity and its damaging health effects. Strategies described in this chapter include screening for food insecurity in families; reviewing services available at national, state, and local levels; and integrating intervention strategies into clinical workflows to alleviate food insecurity and its effects on child health.

Effects of Food Insecurity on Child Health

Nutrition and Obesity

Nutrition deficiencies are more common among children who experience food insecurity. For example, children and adolescents who experience food insecurity are more likely to have iron deficiency[5,6] and preadolescent boys (aged 8–11 years) who experience food insecurity are more likely to have lower bone density as a consequence of malnutrition.[7] The mechanisms through which food insecurity may lead to obesity among children and adolescents are not yet completely clear. But reports highlight that food insecurity and overweight/obesity are often comorbid in childhood.[8,9] Furthermore, food insecurity is more prevalent among populations known to be at increased risk for obesity (eg, lower-income populations, Black and Hispanic children).[10] This may be caused by factors such as systemic racism, economic inequality, and food deserts.[11]

Mental Health, Development, and Academic Outcomes

There is a strong association between experiences of food insecurity and child depression and anxiety.[12] Studies have postulated that food insecurity may influence psychosocial adjustment through its effects on family dynamics, as food insecurity increases parental psychological distress and depression.[13,14] In adolescents, prolonged food insecurity may result in worry, shame, and isolation, which can also trigger chronic stress.[15] Subsequently, this additional chronic stress may result in elevated cortisol levels and maladaptive emotional over-reactivity with long-term consequences for mental health.[15]

Likely because of its effect on mental health, food insecurity is also linked to poorer academic and cognitive outcomes, as well as behavioral conditions and issues such as attention-deficit/hyperactivity disorder and aggression.[16] Food insecurity in children of kindergarten age has been associated with lower academic achievement over the next several years.[16] While food insecurity among school-aged children has been shown to be associated with poorer academic outcomes, food insecurity among adolescents has been linked with mainly psychosocial outcomes. These include depression, anxiety, suicidal ideation, and substance use disorders.[16]

Other Child-Related Outcomes

Food insecurity has also been studied in conjunction with other child health outcomes, including asthma, emergency department (ED) use, and long-term associations with experiencing food insecurity as an adult. Given the detrimental effects of food insecurity on a child's health, it is critical for clinicians to be able to recognize the diverse manifestations of food insecurity among children and their families in the clinical setting.

Key Concept

Food insecurity has been linked to various child health outcomes, including

- **Nutritional deficiencies**
- **Negative impact on mental health and psychosocial development**
- **Poorer academic and cognitive outcomes**
- **High rates of asthma and ED use**

Manifestations of Food Insecurity in Pediatric Clinical Practice

The presence of food insecurity may emerge during a clinical assessment of the child or caregiver or when assessing the household or neighborhood context. **Figure 7-1** describes various manifestations of food insecurity at the child, caregiver, household/family, and neighborhood levels. The development and maintenance of healthy dietary behaviors are the foundation for maintaining healthy growth curves in children. Thus, clinicians regularly conduct dietary assessments during health supervision visits, with more detailed assessments in partnership with a nutritionist if growth abnormalities are detected. Food insecurity may manifest in

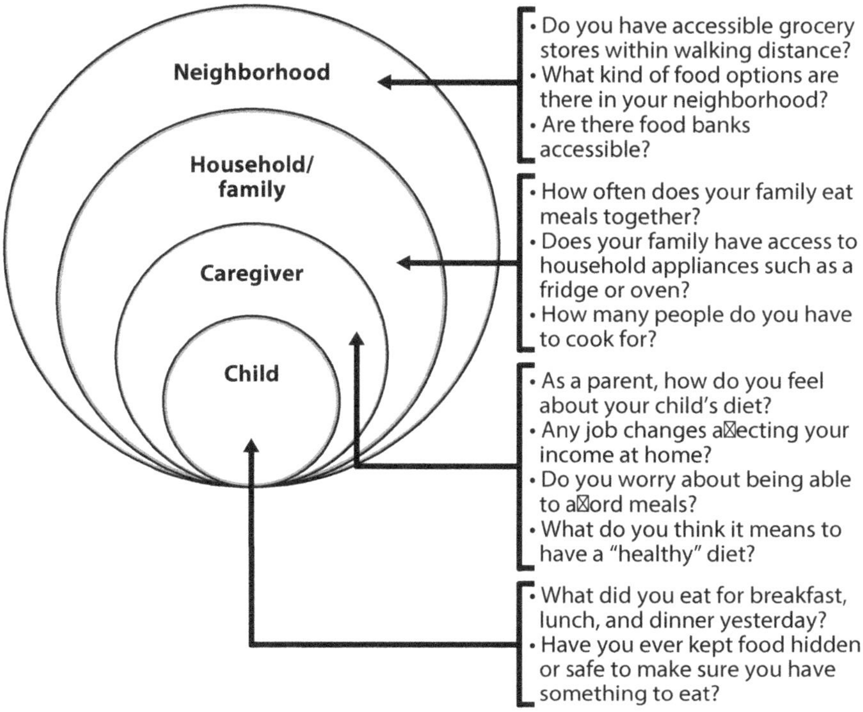

Figure 7-1. Clinical Manifestations of Food Insecurity

various ways that can provide insight into decreased nutritional quality or inadequate food intake.[17] For example, food insecurity may show itself through *diet monotony,* or a diet lacking in diversity, which can occur when there is reluctance to try new foods for fear of food waste. Food insecurity can also show itself as overconsumption of shelf-stable, processed, and energy-dense foods that are less expensive or more convenient. Other behaviors indicative of a history of food insecurity, particularly in the setting of anxiety-related comorbidities, may be food hoarding, food obsessions, or overeating.[18]

Pediatric practitioners must partner with parents and caregivers in the primary care setting to optimize children's health. In doing so, food insecurity may be detected in association with increased parental stress,[13] which can influence parent goal setting and behaviors around child feeding. Parents who experience food insecurity early in their child's life have been found to use less responsive feeding styles that are associated with unhealthy weight gain.[19,20]

When pediatric practitioners acknowledge the broader household and neighborhood context of children's health behaviors, particularly when they suspect food insecurity, there are other comorbid social stressors. These include low health literacy, housing insecurity, and inadequate access to primary care.[21] Furthermore, practitioners should also consider the broader neighborhood context in which families live when delivering recommendations about increasing healthy fruit and vegetable intake. Previously referred to as "food deserts" at the Economic Research Services, there are various factors that define areas considered as low income or low access to health foods (ie, distance to a store, average income of the neighborhood, availability of public transportation).[22] Understanding the food environment allows providers to work together with families to help troubleshoot and plan how to acquire healthy food (refer to the Supplemental Nutrition Assistance Program Benefits section later in this chapter for availability through food delivery). Through the USDA website, pediatric practitioners can use the Food Access Research Atlas[23] to view indicators for food access specific to their clinic's patient population.

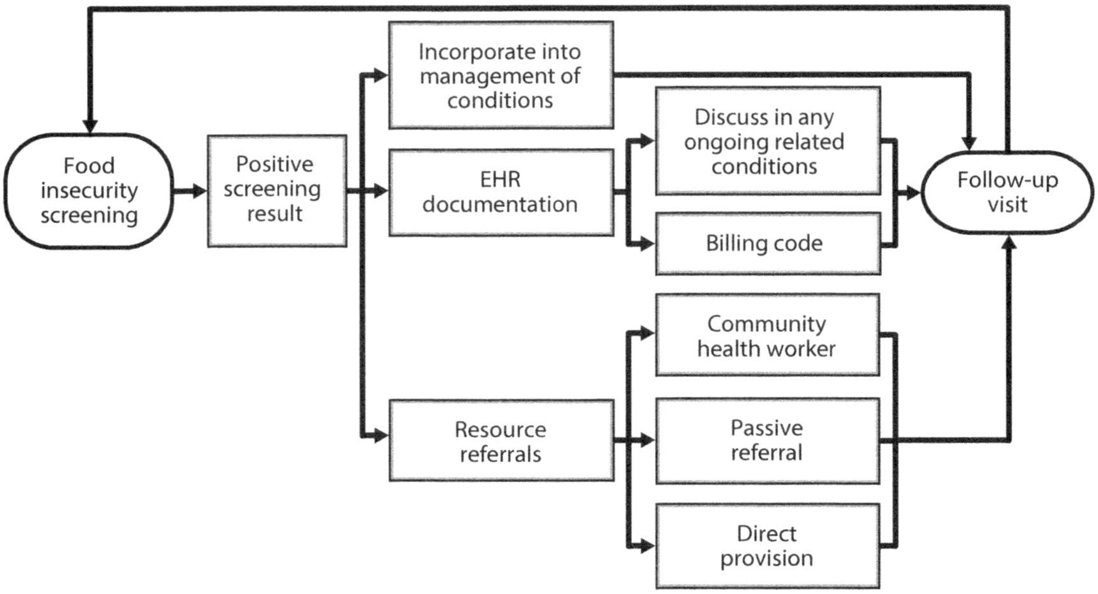

Figure 7-2. Screening for Food Insecurity: A Sample Flowchart
EHR indicates electronic health record.

Screening for Food Insecurity

Physician organizations, including the American Academy of Pediatrics (AAP) and the American Academy of Family Physicians, recommend universal screening for food insecurity.[24] Clinical encounters represent important opportunities for medical staff to screen for social determinants of health (SDOH) within the context of a trusted relationship. This includes both routine visits and any other follow-up visits. Using validated screening tools not only allows primary care systems to more reliably connect families to appropriate community resources but also facilitates clinician discussions with families regarding the impact of food insecurity on health behaviors at home. Finally, documentation of the presence of food insecurity within the patient's health record facilitates continuity of care and ongoing support (**Figure 7-2**).

Key Concept

It is recommended that patients and families be universally screened for food insecurity with a validated screening tool. By implementing universal screening, clinicians can better connect families to appropriate resources and referrals.

The 2-Question Hunger Vital Sign

The Hunger Vital Sign (**Box 7-1**) is a validated food insecurity screening tool endorsed by the AAP and the Center for Medicare & Medicaid Services (CMS), and it has also been incorporated into the Accountable Health Communities screening tool.[25]

Box 7-1.
The Hunger Vital Sign

1. Within the past 12 months, we worried whether our food would run out before we got money to buy more.
2. Within the past 12 months, the food we bought just didn't last and we didn't have money to get more.

From The Hunger Vital Sign. Children's HealthWatch. Accessed May 3, 2024. https://childrenshealthwatch.org/public-policy/hunger-vital-sign.

An affirmative answer to one or both statements is considered a positive screening result for food insecurity. Before the validation of the Hunger Vital Sign, the USDA had a full 18-item question scale assessing food insecurity, which serves as the criterion standard for defining food insecurity. Research has shown, however, that an affirmative response to either Hunger Vital Sign question had a sensitivity of 97% and specificity of 83%, in line with the full 18-question scale. Furthermore, saying yes to either statement was associated with poor child health, increased hospitalizations, and developmental risk, validating the usefulness of the Hunger Vital Sign.[26]

US Department of Agriculture Screening Tool for Food Insufficiency

For clinical settings serving a patient population with a lower prevalence of food insecurity, health care systems may consider using a 1-question screening tool for efficiency. The USDA has a screening tool that can be used as a preliminary screening tool for food insecurity instead of the 2-question screening tool.[27] This question asks, "Which of these statements best describes the food eaten in your household in the last 12 months?" Respondents can answer in one of the following ways:

- *Enough of the kinds of food (I/we) want to eat*
- *Enough, but not always the kinds of food (I/we) want*
- *Sometimes not enough to eat*
- *Often not enough to eat*

Additional Screening Tools

The USDA has a set of screening questionnaires (6-, 10-, and 18-item US Household Food Security Survey Module) that are often used in the research setting to classify household-, parent-, and child-level food insecurity granularly. Food insecurity screening is also often incorporated into other screening tools. For example, a question about food insecurity ("In the past month, was there any day when you or anyone in your family went hungry because you did not have enough money for food?") is already included in the Survey of Well-being of Young Children.[28]

Once a patient or family has been identified as at risk of experiencing food insecurity, clinicians can take the next step by connecting the patient of family to the appropriate resources.

Federal Programs and Local Resources

When families screen positive for food insecurity, primary care systems can refer them to programs and resources at the federal, state, and local levels. Additionally, clinicians can refer to the FRAC *Screen and Intervene* toolkit, which was created in partnership with the AAP to provide key information related to addressing food insecurity in the pediatric setting.[2] When available, engagement of community health workers (CHWs) can be critical in improving access and accessibility to services. Community health workers are trained public health professionals who serve as liaisons between valuable resources and the community. Referral to a CHW has been shown to have improved follow-through in addressing food insecurity needs.[29] In primary care settings without CHWs, clinicians can directly recommend federal, state, and local resources, such as the Special Supplemental Nutrition Program for Women, Infants, and Children; the Supplemental Nutrition Assistance Program; and the National School Lunch Program. **Figure 7-3** depicts the childhood age ranges that each resource supports.

Key Concept

Clinicians can support patients experiencing food insecurity in the following ways:

- **Referring to a CHW when available**
- **Familiarizing themselves with local, state, and federal resources and programs that address food insecurity**
- **Assessing eligibility and connecting patients at risk of experiencing food insecurity to these resources and programs**

Federal Programs

The Special Supplemental Nutrition Program for Women, Infants, and Children

The Special Supplemental Nutrition Program for Women, Infants, and Children (commonly known as WIC) supports the nutrition of families with infants and young children (**Figure 7-3**). The program provides supplemental foods, breastfeeding support, and nutrition education for low-income pregnant, breastfeeding, and non-breastfeeding postpartum women and people, as well as families with infants and children up to age 5 years who are found to be at nutritional risk, based on clinical assessment. According to the USDA in 2020, an estimated 12.5 million people were eligible to receive WIC benefits per month, yet only 6.3 million people participated in the program. In other words, the share of eligible people who participated in WIC was only 50%.[30] Pediatric practitioners can play a critical role in attempting to close this gap by helping families at risk for food insecurity connect to this resource.

Eligibility and Application

Children younger than 5 years qualify for WIC; eligible adult applicants must be pregnant or breastfeeding. Each state sets income eligibility, which is usually between 100% and 185% of the federal poverty threshold.[31] WIC also covers nutritional risk categories that qualify for support. These include common medical problems, such as iron deficiency anemia; milk protein allergy;

Pregnancy	Infancy	☒ Years	School Age	Adolescents

WIC
Age: Pregnant or breastfeeding mothers, infants, children up to age ☒
Eligibility: Income, regardless of immigration status
Benefits: Breastfeeding support, formula, nutrition for breastfeeding and expecting mothers
Notes for pediatricians: Health care provider must sign a medical referral form

SNAP
Age: All ages
Eligibility: Income, only US citizens and certain lawfully present noncitizens
Benefits: EBT cards that can be used in stores or online in order to purchase healthy foods
Notes for pediatricians: For more information, contact your local SNAP o☒ce. Of note, not every retailer in a community will take EBT cards. Familiariz e yourself with which local stores and online grocery delivery services take EBT cards.

School Lunch
Age: School-aged children at participating schools
Eligibility: Income, already enrolled in WIC or SNAP
Benefits: Free or subsidized school lunch and/or breakfast
Notes for pediatricians: The Summer Food Assistance Program provides meals when school is not in session in low-income communities

Figure 7-3. Federal, State, and Local Programs for Families With Food Insecurity
EBT indicates electronic benefits transfer; SNAP, Supplemental Nutrition Assistance Program; and WIC, Special Supplemental Nutrition Program for Women, Infants, and Children.

or any medical reason requiring a specific diet or formula that may present an increased cost barrier to at-risk families. Of note, WIC has no immigration status requirements, so applicants concerned about having specific documentation can receive benefits through WIC.[32] Pediatric practitioners fill out a WIC form available for download online, which the patient can then bring to a local WIC office to apply and immediately begin receiving services.

Benefits

WIC provides applicants who meet eligibility criteria with an electronic benefits transfer (EBT) card, which functions like a debit card and can be used to purchase foods at participating stores. WIC can also supply infant formula, including specialty formula with medical documentation. Additionally, WIC provides nutrition education, access to health care and other social services, and breastfeeding support (eg, peer counseling, lactation consultations, breast pumps) from certified lactation educators. Pediatric practitioners can visit the USDA website (www.fns.usda.gov/wic) or speak with a local WIC representative to better familiarize themselves with state-specific resources and office locations.

Supplemental Nutrition Assistance Program

The Supplemental Nutrition Assistance Program (SNAP), is a US federal program that provides nutrition benefits to low-income individuals and families. Originally known as the Food Stamp Program, its name was changed in 2008 in effort to avoid stigmatizing families that use the service.[33] Like WIC, the program is administered by the USDA Food and Nutrition Service and is supported through local offices that monitor local retail food stores participating in the program. In 2017, an estimated 14.6 million (or 1 in 5) US children participated in SNAP, according to data from the 2018 Survey of Income and Program Participation.[34,35]

Eligibility and Application

Like WIC, eligibility criteria for SNAP are based on household income at a level determined by the applicant's state of residence.[34] This information can be referenced on each individual state's SNAP websites. Unlike WIC, SNAP eligibility is not limited by a child's age. In addition, the Food and Nutrition Act of 2008 limited eligibility for SNAP benefits to adult US citizens and certain lawfully present noncitizens. Children and adolescents younger than 18 years who are noncitizens, however, qualify for SNAP. Families must apply for SNAP in their state of residence by visiting their local SNAP office or the state agency website.

Benefits

Like WIC benefits, SNAP benefits are provided through an EBT card to which monthly benefits are deposited. Benefits can be used for fruits, vegetables, meat, poultry, fish, and dairy products but exclude alcohol and medications. For families with limited access to grocery stores as a result of where they live or limited transportation, pediatric practitioners can advise families that many food stores (including Amazon, one of the largest online national grocery delivery services[36]) now accept SNAP payments online.

National School Lunch Program

The National School Lunch Program is a federally funded resource that supports school lunches for low-income students in both private and public schools in the United States. Meals must meet federal nutrition standards, meaning meals are balanced with whole grains, fruits, and vegetables. Research has shown that students who receive school meals consume more whole grains, milk, fruits, and vegetables than those who bring their lunches from home or do not participate in the program.[37] Participation in the school lunch program has been shown to reduce food insecurity in households by 14% if at least 1 child received free or reduced-price school lunch.[38] Subsequently, studies show that rates of household food insecurity rise during the summer when children do not have access to school meals.[38,39]

Eligibility and Application

Although state and local requirements vary, children overall qualify for the National School Lunch Program depending on household income and family size. Children from families with incomes at or below 130% of the federal poverty threshold are eligible for free meals, and those with incomes at 130% to 185% of the federal poverty threshold are eligible for reduced-price meals.[40] The overlap of benefits between SNAP, WIC, and the National School Lunch Program should be noted by clinicians, because if a child qualifies for one program, they often automatically qualify for other programs. For example, children who receive SNAP or WIC benefits are enrolled in the federally funded Head Start program; children experiencing homelessness also qualify for the program.[35]

In certain areas (eg, New York City), school lunch is available to all children regardless of income, averting the need for potentially stigmatizing screening processes for children who experience food insecurity.[41] In these areas, pediatric practitioners can also encourage all children to participate in school lunch programs to decrease overall stigma around food insecurity.

Local Resources

Local resources include neighborhood- or city-organized efforts to address hunger within the community.

Food Banks

Food banks and soup kitchens are local food distribution centers that aim to meet the needs of people who have difficulty purchasing food on their own. Access to local food banks and soup kitchens varies by community, but families can be directed to Feeding America (www.feedingamerica.org), a nonprofit organization that has a nationwide network of food banks.[42] Most food banks do not have eligibility requirements, and families are eligible regardless of income or immigration status.

Other Local Resources

Local community gardens or farmers markets can also be a source of fresh produce for families with food insecurity, and many accept federal SNAP benefits.

Electronic Health Record Documentation and Billing

The AAP, the Institute for Healthcare Improvement, and the CMS all recommend that health care systems document SDOH such as food insecurity in their electronic health records (EHRs).[43] **Figure 7-2** depicts a suggested clinic workflow for when to best incorporate EHR documentation, which supports clinical capacity to integrate SDOH into clinical practice as described in the Screening for Food Insecurity section earlier in this chapter. Furthermore, training staff to use appropriate and precise terminology in the EHR can drive evaluation and quality improvement, research, and reimbursement around food insecurity.[43] Current *International Classification of*

Diseases, Tenth Revision, Clinical Modification medical billing codes contain codes for broad SDOH, including food insecurity. In addition to documentation of a positive screening result for food insecurity, clinical workflows should incorporate methods of tracking the success of interventions and referrals within the patient's EHR.

Overall, improved documentation can allow for more robust population health data that can guide future interventions targeting food insecurity.

Key Concept

Using standardized terminology when documenting food insecurity within the EHR can improve both individual patient care and overall population health outcomes by enhancing research, population data, and reimbursement for interventions addressing food insecurity.

Future Directions

As our understanding of how families experience food insecurity and its health consequences continues to expand, recommendations of how to approach the issue will evolve. For example, organizations such as the USDA and National Institutes of Health have begun to use the term *food and nutrition security* to mean "consistent and equitable access to healthy, safe, affordable foods essential to optimal health and well-being."[44] Furthermore, although not part of current validated screening methods, assessing neighborhood food access when screening for food insecurity among pediatric patients may become increasingly important, as research has shown that children who live in low-income neighborhoods that lack resources have poorer health outcomes.[45]

As evidence accumulates about effective intervention strategies to alleviate food insecurity and address its adverse effects on health, clinical guidelines will reflect best practices and recommend evidence-based primary care interventions in the clinic. **Table 7-1** highlights clinical screening programs that have had positive impacts. Overall, programs have used the following approaches[46,47]:

- Passive referrals to local food resources
- Active referrals to food resources (eg, CHWs)
- Direct provision of food in the clinic
- Provision of food vouchers (eg, food prescription programs)

Studies of these programs have demonstrated moderately positive results in effective program linkage and use, although evidence of actual increase in fruit and vegetable intake remains limited.

Finally, pediatric practitioners serve as leading child health advocates who also can influence public policy agendas around food and nutrition. Engagement with the local AAP chapter or participation in activities such as AAP Advocacy Day amplifies pediatric advocacy for patients beyond the clinical interventions to ensure continuing support and resources to mitigate food insecurity and its root causes.[48]

Table 7-1. Clinical Programs Addressing Food Insecurity

Program	Type of Program	Evidence-Based Positive Effects
Well Child Care, Evaluation, Community Resources, Advocacy, Referral, Education (WE CARE)[a]	Food insecurity screening of caregivers of children 6 months and younger at health supervision visits	Increased referrals for and enrollment in community services
Keeping Infants Nourished and Developing[b]	Supplementation of formula, direct delivery of education materials, and referrals to community resources	Increased utilization (engagement with health supervision care), including a completed full set of health supervision visits
Medical Tailored Meals[c]	(For adults) Meals customized to the adult's health care needs	Decreased health care utilization of emergency departments and inpatient admissions
Kaiser,[d] ProMedica,[e] and Geisinger[f]	Robust food insecurity screening programs and programs to supply healthy food to patients	Have not published peer-reviewed studies on program impacts

[a] Garg A, Toy S, Tripodis Y, Silverstein M, Freeman E. Addressing social determinants of health at well child care visits: a cluster RCT. *Pediatrics*. 2015;135(2):e296–e304.

[b] Beck AF, Henize AW, Kahn RS, Reiber KL, Young JJ, Klein MD. Forging a pediatric primary care–community partnership to support food-insecure families. *Pediatrics*. 2014;134(2):e564–e571.

[c] Berkowitz SA, Terranova J, Randall L, Cranston K, Waters DB, Hsu J. Association between receipt of a medically tailored meal program and health care use. *JAMA Intern Med*. 2019;179(6):786–793.

[d] Food and nutrition security: supporting access to nutritious food for healthy communities. Kaiser Permanente. Accessed May 3, 2024. https://about.kaiserpermanente.org/content/internet/kp/kpcomms/en/commitments-and-impact/public-policy/our-key-issues/food-and-nutrition-security.html.

[e] Oostra R. Starving for a solution: hunger as a health issue. *ProMedica* blog. Accessed May 3, 2024. https://www.promedica.org/blog/starving-for-a-solution-hunger-as-a-health-issue.

[f] Feinberg AT, Slotkin JR, Hess A, Erskin AR. How Geisinger treats diabetes by giving away free, healthy food. Harvard Business Review. October 25, 2017. Updated December 19, 2017. Accessed May 3, 2024. https://hbr.org/2017/10/how-geisinger-treats-diabetes-by-giving-away-free-healthy-food.

Key Concept

Beyond the clinic setting, clinicians can serve at the forefront of fighting food insecurity through various policy advocacy opportunities.

Key Points

- At least 1 in 7 children experiences food insecurity.
- Children in households with food insecurity are at risk for nutritional problems, increased developmental issues, mental health problems, and poorer overall health.
- Pediatric practitioners are on the frontlines of identifying food insecurity in children and households and being able to intervene at the appropriate time.
- Documenting in the health record whether families experience food insecurity increases clinical capacity to integrate SDOH into medical care through program and resource referrals, as well as to inform panel surveillance of material hardships.
- There are interventions addressing food insecurity at the local, state, and federal levels. Referring patients to these programs can serve as an important step in mitigating the detrimental effects of food insecurity on child health.

References

1. Economic Research Service. Food security in the U.S. US Department of Agriculture. Updated October 25, 2023. Accessed July 11, 2024. https://www.ers.usda.gov/topics/food-nutrition-assistance/food-security-in-the-u-s
2. Ashbrook A, Essel K, Montez K, Bennet-Tejes DB. *Screen and Intervene: A Toolkit for Pediatricians to Address Food Insecurity*. American Academy of Pediatrics, Food Research & Action Center; 2021. Accessed May 3, 2024. https://frac.org/aaptoolkit
3. Parekh N, Ali SH, O'Connor J, et al. Food insecurity among households with children during the COVID-19 pandemic: results from a study among social media users across the United States. *Nutr J*. 2021;20(1):73 PMID: 34461913 doi: 10.1186/s12937-021-00732-2
4. Coleman-Jensen A, Rabbitt MP, Gregory CA, Singh A. *Household Food Security in the United States in 2020*. Economic Research Service, US Dept of Agriculture; 2021. Economic Research Report 298
5. Eicher-Miller HA, Mason AC, Weaver CM, McCabe GP, Boushey CJ. Food insecurity is associated with iron deficiency anemia in US adolescents. *Am J Clin Nutr*. 2009;90(5):1358–1371 PMID: 19776137 doi: 10.3945/ajcn.2009.27886
6. Wu AC, Lesperance L, Bernstein H. Screening for iron deficiency. *Pediatr Rev*. 2002;23(5):171–178 PMID: 11986493 doi: 10.1542/pir.23.5.171
7. Eicher-Miller HA, Mason AC, Weaver CM, McCabe GP, Boushey CJ. Food insecurity is associated with diet and bone mass disparities in early adolescent males but not females in the United States. *J Nutr*. 2011;141(9):1738–1745 PMID: 21795427 doi: 10.3945/jn.111.142059
8. Eisenmann JC, Gundersen C, Lohman BJ, Garasky S, Stewart SD. Is food insecurity related to overweight and obesity in children and adolescents? a summary of studies, 1995–2009. *Obes Rev*. 2011;12(5): e73–e83 PMID: 21382151 doi: 10.1111/j.1467-789X.2010.00820.x
9. Metallinos-Katsaras E, Must A, Gorman K. A longitudinal study of food insecurity on obesity in preschool children. *J Acad Nutr Diet*. 2012;112(12):1949–1958 PMID: 23174682 doi: 10.1016/j.jand.2012.08.031
10. Coleman-Jensen A, Rabbitt MP, Gregory CA, Singh A. *Household Food Security in the United States in 2016*. Economic Research Service, US Dept of Agriculture; 2017. Economic Research Report 237
11. Hunger hits Black communities harder. Feeding America. Accessed October 3, 2024. https://www.feedingamerica.org/hunger-in-america/black-communities
12. Thomas MMC, Miller DP, Morrissey TW. Food insecurity and child health. *Pediatrics*. 2019;144(4): e20190397 PMID: 31501236 doi: 10.1542/peds.2019-0397
13. Berge JM, Fertig AR, Trofholz A, Neumark-Sztainer D, Rogers E, Loth K. Associations between parental stress, parent feeding practices, and child eating behaviors within the context of food insecurity. *Prev Med Rep*. 2020;19:101146 PMID: 32642403 doi: 10.1016/j.pmedr.2020.101146
14. Whitaker RC, Phillips SM, Orzol SM. Food insecurity and the risks of depression and anxiety in mothers and behavior problems in their preschool-aged children. *Pediatrics*. 2006;118(3):e859–e868 PMID: 16950971 doi: 10.1542/peds.2006-0239
15. Dush JL. Adolescent food insecurity: a review of contextual and behavioral factors. *Public Health Nurs*. 2020;37(3):327–338 PMID: 31970826 doi: 10.1111/phn.12708
16. Shankar P, Chung R, Frank DA. Association of food insecurity with children's behavioral, emotional, and academic outcomes: a systematic review. *J Dev Behav Pediatr*. 2017;38(2):135–150 PMID: 28134627 doi: 10.1097/DBP.0000000000000383
17. Morales ME, Berkowitz SA. The relationship between food insecurity, dietary patterns, and obesity. *Curr Nutr Rep*. 2016;5(1):54–60 PMID: 29955440 doi: 10.1007/s13668-016-0153-y

18. Frayn M, Trainor C, Lin M, et al. Patient perceptions of the relationship between food insecurity and eating disorder treatment: a qualitative exploration. *Int J Eat Disord*. 2022;55(3):332–342 PMID: 34971455 doi: 10.1002/eat.23661

19. Almaatani D, Zurbau A, Khoshnevisan F, et al. The association between parents' stress and parental feeding practices and feeding styles: systematic review and meta-analysis of observational studies. *Matern Child Nutr*. 2023;19(1):e13448 PMID: 36284502 doi: 10.1111/mcn.13448

20. Gross RS, Mendelsohn AL, Fierman AH, Racine AD, Messito MJ. Food insecurity and obesogenic maternal infant feeding styles and practices in low-income families. *Pediatrics*. 2012;130(2):254–261 PMID: 22826569 doi: 10.1542/peds.2011-3588

21. Ma CT, Gee L, Kushel MB. Associations between housing instability and food insecurity with health care access in low-income children. *Ambul Pediatr*. 2008;8(1):50–57 PMID: 18191782 doi: 10.1016/j.ambp.2007.08.004

22. Economic Research Services. About the atlas. US Department of Agriculture. Updated April 27, 2021. Accessed June 14, 2024. https://www.ers.usda.gov/data-products/food-access-research-atlas/about-the-atlas

23. Economic Research Service. Go to the atlas. US Department of Agriculture. Updated July 6, 2023. Accessed May 3, 2024. https://www.ers.usda.gov/data-products/food-access-research-atlas/go-to-the-atlas

24. Patil SP, Craven K, Kolasa K. Food insecurity: how you can help your patients. *Am Fam Physician*. 2018;98(3):143–145 PMID: 30215895

25. Billioux A, Verlander K, Anthony S, Alley D. Standardized screening for health-related social needs in clinical settings: the Accountable Health Communities screening tool. National Academy of Medicine. May 30, 2017. Accessed May 3, 2024. https://nam.edu/standardized-screening-for-health-related-social-needs-in-clinical-settings-the-accountable-health-communities-screening-tool

26. The Hunger Vital Sign. Children's HealthWatch. Accessed May 3, 2024. https://childrenshealthwatch.org/public-policy/hunger-vital-sign

27. Economic Research Service. U.S. Household Food Security Survey Module: three-stage design, with screeners. US Department of Agriculture. September 2012. Accessed May 3, 2024. https://www.ers.usda.gov/topics/food-nutrition-assistance/food-security-in-the-u-s/survey-tools/#household

28. Survey of Well-being of Young Children. Age-specific forms. Tufts Medicine. Accessed May 3, 2024. https://pediatrics.tuftsmedicalcenter.org/the-survey-of-wellbeing-of-young-children/age-specific-forms

29. Division of Diabetes Translation, National Center for Chronic Disease Prevention and Health Promotion. The role of community health workers in addressing food and nutrition security and social support during the COVID-19 pandemic. Centers for Disease Control and Prevention. November 2022. Accessed May 3, 2024. https://stacks.cdc.gov/view/cdc/122282

30. Food and Nutrition Service. National and state level estimates of WIC eligibility and program reach in 2020. US Department of Agriculture. Updated November 3, 2023. Accessed May 3, 2024. https://www.fns.usda.gov/wic/eligibility-and-program-reach-estimates-2020

31. Food and Nutrition Service. WIC eligibility requirements. US Department of Agriculture. Updated March 26, 2024. Accessed May 3, 2024. https://www.fns.usda.gov/wic/wic-eligibility-requirements

32. Food and Nutrition Service. WIC program—immigration participation in the WIC program. US Department of Agriculture. Updated June 25, 2024. Accessed July 11, 2024. https://www.fns.usda.gov/wic/immigration-participation

33. Food and Nutrition Service. A short history of SNAP. US Department of Agriculture. Updated December 28, 2023. Accessed May 3, 2024. https://www.fns.usda.gov/snap/short-history-snap

34. Food and Nutrition Service. SNAP eligibility. US Department of Agriculture. Updated April 26, 2024. Accessed May 3, 2024. https://www.fns.usda.gov/snap/recipient/eligibility

35. King MD, Giefer KG. Nearly a third of children who receive SNAP participate in two or more additional programs. US Census Bureau. June 30, 2021. Updated April 12, 2022. Accessed May 3, 2024. https://www.census.gov/library/stories/2021/06/most-children-receiving-snap-get-at-least-one-other-social-safety-net-benefit.html

36. Top 12 food and grocery delivery companies in the US. BuildCentral. Accessed May 3, 2024. https://www.buildcentral.com/top-12-food-and-grocery-delivery-companies-in-the-us

37. School meals. CDC Healthy Schools. Reviewed October 19, 2022. Accessed May 3, 2024. https://www.cdc.gov/healthyschools/nutrition/schoolmeals.htm

38. Huang J, Barnidge E. Low-income children's participation in the National School Lunch Program and household food insufficiency. *Soc Sci Med.* 2016;150:8–14 PMID: 26722983 doi: 10.1016/j.socscimed.2015.12.020

39. Huang J, Barnidge E, Kim Y. Children receiving free or reduced-price school lunch have higher food insufficiency rates in summer. *J Nutr.* 2015;145(9):2161–2168 PMID: 26203095 doi: 10.3945/jn.115.214486

40. School meal eligibility and reimbursements. Food Research & Action Center. Accessed July 11, 2024. https://frac.org/school-meal-eligibility-reimbursements

41. School meals. NYC Public Schools. Accessed July 11, 2024. https://www.schools.nyc.gov/school-life/food/school-meals

42. Find your local food bank. Feeding America. Accessed May 3, 2024. https://www.feedingamerica.org/find-your-local-foodbank

43. *ICD-10.* Centers for Medicare & Medicaid Services. Accessed October 8, 2024. https://www.cms.gov/medicare/coding-billing/icd-10-codes

44. Food and nutrition security. US Department of Agriculture. Accessed May 3, 2024. https://www.usda.gov/nutrition-security

45. Morrissey TW, Oellerich D, Meade E, Simms J, Stock A. Neighborhood poverty and children's food insecurity. *Child Youth Serv Rev.* 2016;66:85–93 doi: 10.1016/j.childyouth.2016.05.006

46. De Marchis EH, Torres JM, Benesch T, et al. Interventions addressing food insecurity in health care settings: a systematic review. *Ann Fam Med.* 2019;17(5):436–447 PMID: 31501207 doi: 10.1370/afm.2412

47. McKay FH, Spiteri S, Zinga J, et al. Systematic review of interventions addressing food insecurity in pregnant women and new mothers. *Curr Nutr Rep.* 2022;11(3):486–499 PMID: 35501553 doi: 10.1007/s13668-022-00418-z

48. Hartline-Grafton H, Hassink SG. Food insecurity and health: practices and policies to address food insecurity among children. *Acad Pediatr.* 2021;21(2):205–210 PMID: 32653691 doi: 10.1016/j.acap.2020.07.006

CHAPTER 8

Social Care Interventions

Michael J. Luke, MD

Health systems interested in screening for health-related social needs must first ensure they are equipped with accessible and family-centered intervention strategies to address any identified needs. Several factors, such as variability in severity of need among families and differences in resource availability based on geography, serve as considerable barriers to designing and streamlining social needs interventions. Some common strategies used in health care to overcome these barriers and address families' needs include aggregated resource lists, in-person support to navigate these resources, and partnerships with community organizations that can offer resources directly. Over time, more and more creative models have been developed to address specific social need domains, which can serve as examples for any health system interested in designing its own interventions. Given the increasing overlap between medical and social care complexity in pediatric care, continued collaborative, family-centered, and community-engaged approaches will be critical to achieve health equity.

CHAPTER 8

Social Care Interventions

Michael J. Luke, MD

Although health systems are increasingly recognizing the importance of the social drivers of health (SDOH) in clinical care, not all clinical settings are equipped to address the individual-level social and economic needs that affect patients' health. These needs are often referred to as *health-related social needs* (HRSNs) and include concerns such as homelessness or lack of access to food. In this chapter, we explore a general approach to assist families with their HRSNs, offer common strategies to support families in the health care setting or in the community, and share examples of select evidence-based interventions to address specific HRSNs.

General Considerations for Social Care Interventions

Essential Characteristics for Social Care Interventions

Given the potentially sensitive nature of HRSNs, many guiding principles and best practices have been recommended to ensure that a family-centered approach is used in addressing them. While exploring the SDOH has become routine practice in providing holistic pediatric care, there is a delicate balance between asking patients questions to best understand their social contexts, so one can offer appropriate care, and diving deep into potentially intimate life struggles. For additional guidance on striking this balance, refer to the Training Health Care Staff Members section of Chapter 4, Screening for Social Needs in the Clinical Setting.

Advocates for high-value care implore that clinicians abstain from unnecessary medical tests that would not change their medical decision-making. As such, scholars of the SDOH have emphasized that if providers choose to explore patients' HRSNs, such as through HRSN screening, they should be prepared to act on the results with appropriate interventions. As discussed throughout Chapter 4, trust between the family and provider has been shown to be critical in ensuring successful health care delivery, especially in longitudinal models such as primary care. Therefore, providers should consider the potentially unintended consequences on the patient-physician relationship if they do not meet families' expectations for support.[1]

What dictates whether an intervention activity is appropriate? While no formal guidelines have been established, ideal approaches to addressing social needs should be reasonable, accessible, strengths based, family centered, and culturally competent. Here we will highlight these essential characteristics for all social intervention strategies.

First, resources should not only be available but also be practically reasonable and attainable solutions to families' needs. For example, public transportation reimbursement may be helpful for many families with transportation barriers but not for a family with a child whose medically complex condition requires ambulance transport to clinic visits.

Strengths-based approaches have been highlighted as successful ways to care for unique populations, so leveraging a strengths-based model to discuss their HRSNs and how these needs can be overcome may offer comfort to these families and help preserve and even strengthen the provider-family relationship.[2]

A hallmark of pediatric care delivery is the family-centered approach. As with all other aspects of pediatric care, patient and family buy-in is crucial to success. When exploring assistance options for families, collaborating with caregivers to discover options they feel comfortable with pursuing is of immense value.[3] Similarly, just as in all aspects of care, offering culturally competent recommendations can ensure that intervention activities are in congruence with families' ways of life. For example, providing a referral to a faith-based support group may not be appropriate for a patient with religious trauma.

Key Concept

When considering an assistance strategy for families with identified social needs, providers should ensure that all recommendations are reasonable, accessible, strengths based, family centered, and culturally competent.

Common Barriers to Intervention Strategies

Although the importance of the SDOH has been recognized for decades, there are still barriers to robust HRSN interventions (refer to the Barriers to Screening section of Chapter 4, Screening for Social Needs in the Pediatric Clinical Setting). While several organizations, including the American Academy of Pediatrics (AAP), recommend screening for and addressing HRSNs, there is no standardized approach that has been identified. That is partly because pediatric scholarship in this area remains in its early stages. More importantly, however, it is challenging to standardize interventions at a national level when resources vary widely both by region and over time.[4] Welfare programs are often state specific, including their availability, eligibility, and enrollment processes, and community-based organizations (CBOs) vary from state to state. Additionally, resources fluctuate over time, often influenced by policy changes and major events, such as in the wake of the 2020 global pandemic, when there were significant temporary changes in government-based and community-organized resources available.[5]

Key Concept

Standardizing intervention strategies to address HRSNs remains a critical challenge in health care, as government- and community-based resources vary significantly across states and over time.

Another barrier to implementing assistance activities is identifying the amount of support that families need. Studies have shown that families' expectations for social support is highly variable, ranging from no assistance to frequent follow-up with a care navigator. Research suggests that higher intervention dosages that involved more frequent check-ins with families by navigators led to more success addressing unmet needs.[6] Therefore, to provide optimal care, health systems should build interventions that are customizable and have the infrastructure to offer extensive support if needed. This topic is covered more in the Modality of Screening section of Chapter 4.

Creating comprehensive social support infrastructure requires investment, and a limiting factor is that historically, health care funding to address HRSNs has been low. This is in part caused by a lack of financial incentives for health systems to address them. This will, however, change in time. In 2019, the National Academy of Sciences published a report calling for social care to be integrated into health care delivery, and in 2022, following the SARS-CoV-2 pandemic, the Quintuple Aim for health care improvement was established to nationally prioritize the advancement of health equity. Subsequently in 2023, several regulatory bodies, including the National Committee for Quality Assurance, The Joint Commission, and the Centers for Medicare & Medicaid Services, released new requirements and quality measures related to HRSN screening and intervention for health plans and health systems. Thus, the desire to meet these quality expectations, as well as future expansions in insurance coverage and value-based methods for reimbursement, will likely incentivize funding for more social care interventions.[7]

Evaluation Approaches for Social Care Interventions

As institutions create strategies to address HRSNs, it is imperative to establish key methods for evaluating the efficacy of these interventions. **Figure 8-1** depicts a model framework to guide health centers in the evaluation of their social interventions.[5]

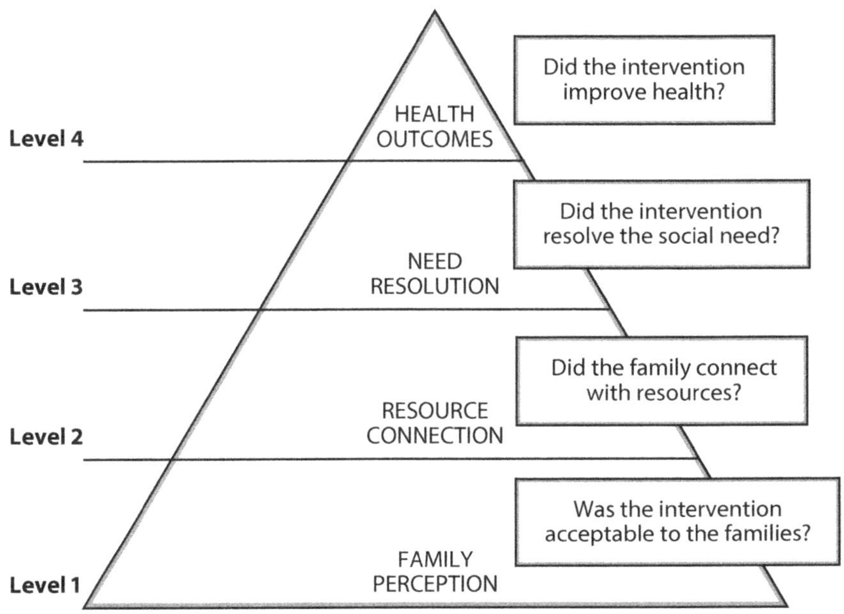

Figure 8-1. Evaluation Model for Health System–Based Social Care Interventions

From Luke MJ, Vasan A. From incentives to outcomes: a framework to implement and evaluate social needs interventions. *Hosp Pediatr.* 2023;13(10):e295–e298.

Interventions to address identified HRSNs should meet 4 primary goals: they should be supported by families, allow for feasible linkage to resources, lead to resolution of identified HRSNs, and, ultimately, result in improved health or reduced health costs. Although there is growing literature exploring caregiver perspectives of screening and responses,[6,8] more research is warranted to explore the efficacy of HRSN interventions on achieving these other key outcome measures. Given the chronic nature of SDOH, current social care interventions could take years or even decades to result in noticeable positive impacts on child health. Therefore, as health centers implement HRSN interventions, it is critical to focus on key process measures, such as resource connection and need resolution, before the ultimate goal of improved health can be achieved.

Key Concept

New interventions designed to address HRSNs should be evaluated to ensure they

1. **Are supported by families**
2. **Allow for feasible linkage to resources**
3. **Lead to resolution of identified HRSNs**
4. **Result in improved health outcomes**

Types of Resources

Resources to address HRSNs typically fall into 3 primary categories based on whether they are managed by the health system, the community, or the government. Health systems can offer a broad range of self-funded services in alignment with their mission or as part of grant initiatives. Although referrals to resources in this category are often easier to make and monitor, as they require only internal coordination, they can be limited in geographic accessibility and can require heavy financial investment on the part of the health system.

Resources managed by the community often include those arranged by CBOs, religious institutions, or other local nonprofit efforts. These also often have geographic limitations. Additionally, it can be challenging for health systems to maintain an updated database of available community resources and track whether families have successfully accessed them.

Finally, government-funded public programs can offer reliable resources with more transparent eligibility but may vary regionally and often have challenging administrative burdens for enrollment.[8] Strategies for assistance should consider these factors when compiling these resources to address identified HRSNs.

Common Social Care Interventions for General Needs

Resource Lists

Identifying local resources can be challenging, especially for families with language barriers or limited access to the internet. To ease this burden, one model that health systems have used is an aggregated list of resources that is available in the local community. This list is often manually collated by health care staff and distributed to families as patient handouts, in their health visit paperwork through electronic health record (EHR) integration, via email, QR code access, or patient portal message. Aggregated resource lists are a low-cost strategy that offers the ability to customize resources for a specific population or need and have been shown to be just as efficacious as in-person longitudinal navigation services in one study, although further research is needed.[9] They can, however, require substantial manual effort up front to input all the resources, as well as continued work to maintain an updated list. And there is the risk of including outdated resource information.

Online Directories

An alternative strategy is to use an online directory that can be searched by zip code. There are several online platforms available that allow users to navigate aggregated, geocoded resources and facilitate referrals to resources and organizations.[10] While some are free access, others carry subscription costs. Additionally, some are patient facing, through which families can search resources themselves on their personal networks, offering flexibility and family autonomy. Others are accessible only by designated users, requiring providers to compile relevant geocoded resources and provide them to patients, which may be preferred by families with barriers to technology use. Some platforms also offer the ability for integration into the EHR for ease of use and the option to have the website text or specific lists translated into select languages other than English.

Key Concept

Practical factors that health systems should consider when creating an intervention to address social needs include the cost of the resource, its adaptability to support families with different levels of need, its accessibility for families with barriers to care, and its accuracy over time and for families regardless of residence.

In-Person Support

With the increased incorporation of SDOH into undergraduate and graduate medical education, health care professionals are becoming more apt to address HRSNs, especially in low-resource settings. There are a variety of health care professionals, however, who offer unique skills and expertise to address certain HRSNs that may be valuable in the primary care setting.

Social Work

Social work consultation is the most common form of HRSN intervention in health care settings across the country.[11] Medical social workers offer a wealth of value to a clinical care team and unique contributions depending on their level of training. In the United States, social workers with a bachelor of social work (BSW) have completed a 4-year undergraduate degree and can join entry-level positions often designated for service-related tasks such as discharge planning and care navigation. Those with a master of social work (MSW) complete a 2-year graduate degree with additional clinical exposure hours and are eligible to become a licensed clinical social worker. As a result, MSWs are eligible to take on clinical social work roles, including offering more extensive social support navigation and providing psychotherapy.[12]

Social workers offer flexibility in social care delivery, as they can be accessible in person or virtually, and since they serve a relatively ubiquitous role, their titles are often quite familiar to families. But this support requires notable financial investment, as those with their MSW degree often earn more than those with their BSW degree. It is unfortunate, though, that given the continued increasing prevalence of HRSNs and mental health conditions, there continues to be limited availability of social workers nationally.[13]

Care Management and Case Management

Families that have children with medically complex conditions often have increased and unique needs related to social supports and care navigation when compared with the general pediatric population.[8] Care management programs, typically led by those with nursing expertise, can often offer these families clinical care navigation and some degree of social support.[14]

Case management offers coordination and advocacy for services to address families' health needs, which may include social barriers such as health costs and transportation. While case management provides temporary service over a specific period, care management offers similar services more longitudinally, beyond any particular clinical encounter or care setting. Given the growing evidence to suggest the need for longitudinal care to address social needs,[6,8] children with medical and social complexity would likely benefit from more care management models.

Key Concept

Given the known association between medical and social complexity in pediatrics, care management serves a critical role in addressing adverse SDOH. Case managers can provide temporary service during a particular clinical encounter or care setting, while care managers typically offer services longitudinally.

Mental Health Support

With the increasing incidence of mental health conditions nationally, there continues to be a need for dedicated mental health support. To address this need, many clinical offices have employed an on-site or virtual psychologist to offer individualized therapy, mental health resources, and referrals to a psychiatrist.

Given the long-standing issues of access to psychiatric care, psychologists often function as a bridge to more advanced care, offering lifestyle counseling and brief behavior intervention strategies while psychiatric referrals are in process. This approach does not, however, undermine the importance of psychiatric care, as psychologists are unable to pharmacologically manage mental health conditions, and the combination of therapy and medication has been shown to be the most efficacious in managing several psychiatric diagnoses. Additionally, there are unique limitations in pediatric practices, as psychologists are unable to offer reimbursable counseling directly to caregivers with identified mental health concerns unless those caregivers are also registered to the practice.[15]

Community Health Work

Structural racism and prejudice have led many marginalized communities, which share a disproportionate burden of HRSNs, to distrust the health care system. This has been a particular challenge for designing and executing effective social care interventions for these families. Community health workers (CHWs) have offered a promising solution to this challenge by acting as a sociocultural bridge between health care systems and the communities they serve. They have strong ties to the community with additional health care–related training, often involving a certification, and thus offer immense value as liaisons in both volunteer and paid capacities. In addition, they serve a variety of functional roles with various titles, including, but not limited to, patient advocates, care navigators, peer advisers, health ambassadors, or, in Spanish-speaking communities, promotoras de salud (promoters of health).[16,17] These roles can be served in the clinical setting or in the community, including in patients' homes.

Community health workers offer a community-centered approach and can reduce stigma associated with social needs intervention while providing job opportunities to members in the community. There is substantial evidence to support the use of CHWs to assist with identified HRSNs, and while their scope of practice varies, further research will likely elucidate the potential of their contributions across health care settings.

Partnerships

An alternative strategy to address HRSNs is to leverage existing infrastructure and expertise in the surrounding community by forming partnerships. Partnerships can be informal, involving a verbal understanding of mutual benefit for a common shared goal, or formal, involving a contract.

Medical-Legal Partnerships

Many HRSNs can be addressed through legal remedies. As such, medical-legal partnerships (MLPs) have been established to facilitate easy access to legal services for families with identified needs. The SDOH that are most associated with legal needs include income, housing and utilities, education and employment, legal status, and personal and family stability (I-HELP), as outlined in **Figure 8-2**. Medical-legal partnerships have been shown to have several benefits for patients and families, including improved treatment of chronic disease, most notably asthma and sickle cell disease; medical care engagement; and stress reduction.[18] Furthermore, MLPs may offer additional benefits to health care staff, including improved education on health-related legal issues and provision of resources to integrate into the EHR.[18] The National Center for Medical-Legal Partnership also maintains a free-access online toolkit for providers interested in forming partnerships with their own health care facilities.

Medical-Financial Partnerships

Financial stress associated with poverty has been linked with poor health outcomes. Therefore, to better integrate financial and clinical interventions to improve families' overall health, some health systems have established a medical-financial partnership (MFP) as a new care modality. Support including free tax preparation, financial coaching, matched savings programs, and employment assistance has been shown to improve financial stability for families and reduce their risk for poverty, with positive impacts on children's health. Models for MFPs include complete on-site financial services with case management, tailored on-site financial services, and referrals for off-site financial services, as diagrammed in **Figure 8-3**.[19] To learn more about families facing financial stress and ways to support them, refer to Chapter 5, Financial Assistance and Access to Care.

I-HELP® Issue	Civil Legal Aid Interventions	Related Social Determinant of Health	Impact on Health / Health Care Talking Points
Income	**Benefits Unit:** Appeal denials of food stamps, health insurance, cash benefits, and disability benefits	Increase the availability of resources to meet daily basic needs	1. Increasing someone's income means s/he makes fewer trade-offs between affording food and health care, including medications. 2. Being able to afford enough healthy food helps people manage chronic diseases and helps children grow and develop.
Housing & utilities	**Housing Unit:** Secure housing subsidies; Improve substandard conditions; Prevent eviction; Protect against utility shut-off	Ensure healthy physical environments	1. A stable, decent, affordable home helps individuals avoid costly emergency room visits related to homelessness. 2. Consistent housing, heat and electricity helps people follow their medical treatment plans.
Education & Employment	**Education & Employment Units:** Secure specialized education services; Prevent and remedy employment discrimination and enforce workplace rights	Create equal access to the opportunity to learn and work	1. A quality education is the single greatest predictor of a person's adult health. 2. Consistent employment helps provide money for food and safe housing, which also helps avoid costly emergency health care services. 3. Health insurance is often linked to employment.
Legal Status	**Veterans & Immigration Units:** Resolve veteran discharge status; Clear criminal / credit histories; Assist with asylum applications	Create equal access to the opportunity to work	1. Clearing a person's criminal history or helping a veteran change their discharge status helps make consistent employment and access to public benefits possible. 2. Consistent employment provides money for food and safe housing, which helps people avoid costly emergency health care services.
Personal Stability	**Family Law Unit:** Secure restraining orders for domestic violence; Secure adoption, custody and guardianship for children	Reduce exposure to violence and create a safe and healthy community	1. Less violence at home means less need for costly emergency health care services. 2. Stable family relationships significantly reduce stress and allow for better decision-making, including decisions related to health care.

Figure 8-2. Social Issues Associated With Legal Needs (I-HELP)

Reprinted with permission from Marple K. *Framing Legal Care as Health Care*. National Center for Medical-Legal Partnership, Milken Institute School of Public Health, George Washington University; 2015. Accessed September 25, 2024. https://medical-legalpartnership.org/wp-content/uploads/2015/01/Framing-Legal-Care-as-Health-Care-Messaging-Guide.pdf.

Community Partnerships

Community partnerships offer many benefits in addressing HRSNs. These partnerships have classically been associated with CBOs but can also include educational centers, faith-based organizations, housing and transportation agencies, public health departments, local businesses, or service organizations.[20] These partners often support the same communities with similar goals, so partnership provides the ability to align initiatives to reduce duplicate efforts, pool resources to optimize financial expenditure, and strengthen ties and trust between the health system and community. Community partnerships can vary in their degree of structure, ranging from loose affiliations that may simply involve knowledge sharing to more formalized partnerships such as joint contractual ventures, as seen on the spectrum in **Figure 8-4**. Similarly, the degree of

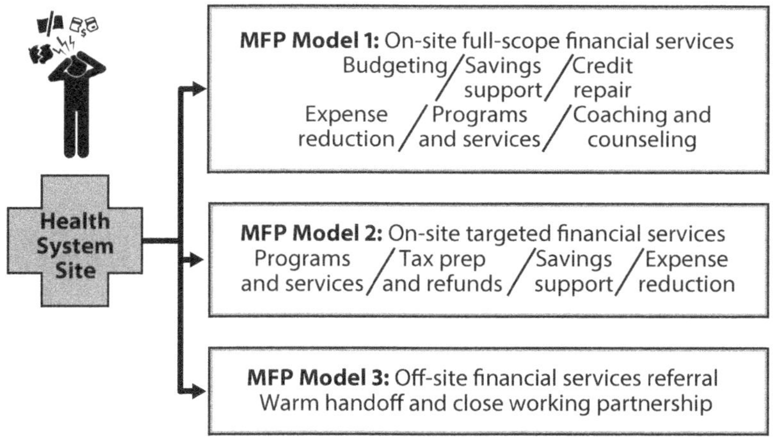

Figure 8-3. Medical-Financial Partnership Models

MFP indicates medical-financial partnership.

Modified with permission from Bell ON, Hole MK, Johnson K, Marcil LE, Solomon BS, Schickedanz A. Medical-financial partnerships: cross-sector collaborations between medical and financial services to improve health. *Acad Pediatr.* 2020;20(2):166–174.

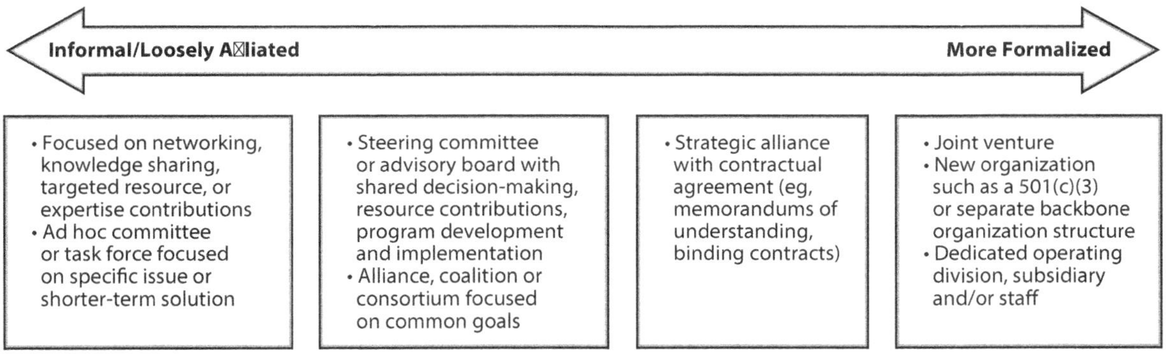

Figure 8-4. Range of Health System–Community Partnership Structures

From *Creating Effective Hospital Community Partnerships to Build a Culture of Health.* Health Research & Educational Trust; 2016:16. Accessed August 1, 2024. http://www.hpoe.org/Reports-HPOE/2016/creating-effective-hospital-community-partnerships.pdf.

services provided by community partners varies and can include a communication line to share updated resource availability, expedited referral pathways for certain community-based services, or even colocation of community partners at clinical sites to allow easy access for patients.

Key Concept

Community partnerships allow health systems to avoid duplicate efforts, pool resources to minimize financial costs, and build stronger relationships between the health system and its surrounding community.

Example Interventions for Specific Needs

There have been several novel initiatives to address HRSNs through health care. Here we will highlight a select few. Although these examples have offered benefits in certain communities, further research may be required to ensure they can be adapted and implemented successfully in different clinical environments.

Economic Stability

Financial Security

Poverty places families at risk for a number of HRSNs. As a result, financial support is thought to be a promising upstream intervention to address many of these needs. Assistance with tax preparation is one potential method of providing financial support by ensuring families access to all available refunds, such as the Earned Income Tax Credit. New York City Health + Hospitals partnered with the New York City Department of Consumer and Worker Protection and 2 CBOs called Urban Upbound and Grow Brooklyn to place free Volunteer Income Tax Assistance–certified services at inpatient and outpatient clinical sites. This program facilitated the filing of greater than 1,000 tax returns during a single tax season and was found to have a favorable return on investment.[21]

Food Access

Food pharmacies were designed to improve access to healthy foods and integrate nutrition support into health care delivery by embracing the concept that food is medicine. This umbrella term can refer to several health care–based strategies. One popular example is a health center–based produce market, which improves access to healthy foods for community members, supports local farmers, and makes space for community engagement. Pennsylvania State Hershey Medical Center created such a market in 2010. Before implementation, the designers collected information from community members on culturally relevant produce needs, from organizers of local farmers markets on potential vendors, and from local government and medical center leadership on fiscal and zoning considerations. They then built a market-governing association to coordinate vendors and regulate fee structure and hours and advertised the market to their employees and local community. Once established, their market served as a source of fresh produce for the community, as well as a venue to distribute public health information.[22]

Education Access and Quality

Education

Early childhood education centers were established to address disparities in learning and development, particularly for youth in low-income families. These programs offer preschool center–based programming to foster cognitive and social growth in children at risk for developmental delay before kindergarten. The longest studied example is the Perry Preschool Project, which was conducted in Ypsilanti, MI, starting in 1962. This program involved preschool education for children aged 3 to 5 years, home visits to offer parenting guidance, and monthly parent group meetings. Although the program did not show a significant impact in intelligence in later childhood, there have been documented benefits to health and economic success decades into the future. Since its launch, several other comparable early childhood education centers have been developed, including The Carolina Abecedarian Project and the Head Start Program, and more work is required to optimize the quality of such programming to ensure the greatest impact.[23]

Literacy

Reading aloud to children with serve-and-return interactions has been shown to positively influence their neurocognitive and socioemotional functioning, later school performance, and career development. In 1989, to capitalize on this, the Reach Out and Read program was established to include books in health supervision visits for children aged 6 months to 5 years to encourage literacy in the clinical setting. (The program has since been expanded to include children from birth to 5 years of age.) Clinic sites interested in participating complete an application, fund the cost of desired books, and have their providers complete training. In 2015, Children's Hospital Colorado implemented the program in their pediatric clinic for Down syndrome. The first published research to explore a literacy intervention program for children with developmental disabilities, this study showed that children with Down syndrome attained independent reading skills comparable to those of children their age without Down syndrome when given the appropriate resources.[24]

Health Care Access and Quality

Primary Care Access

School-based health centers were first developed in the 1960s to improve access to health care for children, and they have continued to grow and evolve. They can be located within or adjacent to an educational institution and offer primary care services, as well as occasionally offer mental, dental, or vision health services. They staff pediatricians, nurses, and medical assistants but often also include social workers and advanced practice providers. As many studies across the country have shown the benefits of preventive care delivery, in light of an increasing mental health burden, Mary's Center in Washington, DC, created a school-based mental health program to build on the successes of school-based health centers and provide on-site behavioral assessments and treatments for children in elementary, middle, and high schools.[25]

Communication

Navigating the health care system can be challenging, especially for families of color that have low incomes, as they disproportionately face health literacy and language barriers. Care navigation is one strategy that has proven to be helpful in clinical settings, as communication barriers can be a significant hindrance to managing chronic medical conditions and addressing HRSNs. One approach implemented at Seattle Children's Hospital in Washington is the Family Bridge Program, which is an inpatient navigation program designed for children of color and their caregivers when the family has low income. The enrolled families were connected to a bilingual guide who would provide the family with education about the hospital, assess for social needs and communication barriers, and offer guidance and emotional support during and shortly after a hospital stay.[26]

Neighborhood and Built Environment

Transportation

Transportation barriers have been associated with missed clinical appointments and poor chronic disease management. Cost-benefit analyses have shown that coverage for non-emergent medical transportation is cost effective for different medical conditions. As such, Boston Medical Center's Pediatric Hematology Clinic funded rideshare services for caregivers of patients with sickle cell disease who endorsed transportation difficulties and then found a significant decrease in no-show rates at a relatively low cost. To create the program, the clinic leveraged an existing relationship between its institution and Uber Health and created a clinic-specific account.

Caregivers were asked about travel access during standard appointment reminder calls, and those who endorsed transportation concerns received funded round-trip rides to their appointments, paid for at market prices.[27]

Housing

Housing remains a frequent source of unmet social needs across the country, including homelessness, housing instability, housing affordability, and poor housing quality. This is of particular interest, as housing quality has been identified as a key social driver for certain pediatric conditions, including asthma, which stands as the most common physical chronic condition among children. To address this, the Children's Hospital of Philadelphia in Pennsylvania designed the Community Asthma Prevention Program Plus Home Repairs in partnership with home repair agencies called Rebuilding Together Philadelphia and the Philadelphia Housing Development Corporation to provide structural repairs to the homes of local children with a history of significant asthma exacerbations. These repairs led to a reduction in known allergens including pests, mold, and dust; decreased reports of asthma-related symptoms; and improvements to families' quality of life.[28,29]

Social and Community Context

Community Violence

Over time, firearm-related injuries have become the number one leading cause of death in children and adolescents. While the AAP continues to advocate for policy change to reduce this incidence, several health care–based strategies have been implemented to help address the firearm epidemic. One notable example has been violence interruption programs, such as hospital-based violence intervention programs, which were designed to engage with people who survived violent trauma to mitigate potential adverse outcomes, including recurrent or retaliatory violence. The details of these programs vary, including eligible age ranges for enrollment; whether staffing includes case managers, social workers, or community representatives; and the degree of partnership with CBOs. One program, called Caught in the Crossfire in Oakland, CA, established in partnership with an organization called Youth ALIVE!, involves peer-based mentoring that begins when the youth is an inpatient, including risk assessment, intensive case management services, and referrals to address HRSNs.[30]

Civic Engagement

Civic participation is recognized as an SDOH. Young adults, especially from racial and ethnic groups that have been marginalized, often have the lowest rates of voter turnout in presidential elections. This turnout is likely in part caused by structural barriers related to the SDOH, such as work schedules and transportation issues. Several health care–based initiatives have been developed to promote civic engagement in these patient populations, including providing easy access to voter registration instructions. One nonprofit organization called Vot-ER implemented a national program to allow health care workers in different pediatric settings to promote civic engagement among their patients by wearing badges with QR codes that link to voter registration.[31]

Future Directions

As the interplay between medical and social complexity continues to grow in pediatrics, it is imperative that we continue to establish collaborative, family-centered, and community-engaged interventions to address HRSNs. As standardized HRSN screening continues to expand, pediatricians must ensure that their health care settings are equipped to address their patients' needs once identified. Further research is needed to identify optimal approaches to improve rates of resource connection for families in need regardless of social and structural barriers, resolve the adverse social conditions contributing to poor health, and, ultimately, reduce disparities in health outcomes.

Key Points

- Providers should ensure all assistance strategies offered to families with HRSNs are reasonable, accessible, strengths based, family centered, and culturally competent.
- Resources to address HRSNs can be divided by whether they are managed by a health system, the community, or the government.
- Social intervention strategies cannot be easily standardized across all health care settings, as resources vary considerably across regions and with time.
- Families have different levels of need and require different degrees of support, so assistance mechanisms must be customizable to provide more extensive support if needed.
- Social intervention strategies should be evaluated to ensure they are supported by families, allow for feasible linkage to resources, lead to resolution of identified HRSNs, and lead to improved health.
- Common intervention strategies to address HRSNs include aggregated resource lists; in-person support, such as from social workers, care managers, or CHWs; and community partnerships.
- Successful interventions to address HRSNs may serve as promising models that must be adapted to fit any new clinical environment and appropriately evaluated for efficacy.

References

1. Garg A, Boynton-Jarrett R, Dworkin PH. Avoiding the unintended consequences of screening for social determinants of health. *JAMA*. 2016;316(8):813–814 PMID: 27367226 doi: 10.1001/jama.2016.9282
2. Bryant J, Bolt R, Botfield JR, et al. Beyond deficit: "strengths-based approaches" in Indigenous health research. *Sociol Health Illn*. 2021;43(6):1405–1421 PMID: 34145599 doi: 10.1111/1467-9566.13311
3. Bouchelle Z, Vasan A. Promoting health equity through family-centered social needs screening and intervention in the inpatient setting. *Hosp Pediatr*. 2022;12(8):e275–e277 PMID: 35843956 doi: 10.1542/hpeds.2022-006725
4. Gottlieb LM, Wing H, Adler NE. A systematic review of interventions on patients' social and economic needs. *Am J Prev Med*. 2017;53(5):719–729 PMID: 28688725 doi: 10.1016/j.amepre.2017.05.011
5. Luke MJ, Vasan A. From incentives to outcomes: a framework to implement and evaluate social needs interventions. *Hosp Pediatr*. 2023;13(10):e295–e298 PMID: 37718960 doi: 10.1542/hpeds.2023-007375
6. Luke MJ, Fernandes DM, Leon Rodriguez F, Acholonu RG, Fiori K. Caregiver perspectives on social needs screening and interventions in an urban children's hospital. *Hosp Pediatr*. 2023;13(8):670–681 PMID: 37483130 doi: 10.1542/hpeds.2022-006736
7. Gottlieb LM, DeSilvey SC, Fichtenberg C, Bernheim S, Peltz A. Developing national social care standards. *Health Affairs Forefront* blog. February 22, 2023. Accessed October 4, 2024. https://www.healthaffairs.org/content/forefront/developing-national-social-care-standards
8. Vasan A, Darko O, Fortin K, Scribano PV, Kenyon CC. Community resource connection for pediatric caregivers with unmet social needs: a qualitative study. *Acad Pediatr*. 2022;22(3):461–469 PMID: 34571255 doi: 10.1016/j.acap.2021.09.010

9. Gottlieb LM, Adler NE, Wing H, et al. Effects of in-person assistance vs personalized written resources about social services on household social risks and child and caregiver health: a randomized clinical trial. *JAMA Netw Open*. 2020;3(3):e200701 PMID: 32154888 doi: 10.1001/jamanetworkopen.2020.0701
10. Lindau ST, Makelarski JA, Abramsohn EM, et al. CommunityRx: a real-world controlled clinical trial of a scalable, low-intensity community resource referral intervention. *Am J Public Health*. 2019;109(4):600–606 PMID: 30789775 doi: 10.2105/ajph.2018.304905
11. Kreuter MW, Thompson T, McQueen A, Garg R. Addressing social needs in health care settings: evidence, challenges, and opportunities for public health. *Annu Rev Public Health*. 2021;42:329–344 PMID: 33326298 doi: 10.1146/annurev-publhealth-090419-102204
12. Grant DM, Toh JS. Medical social work positions: BSW or MSW? *Soc Work Health Care*. 2017;56(4):215–226 PMID: 28271968 doi: 10.1080/00981389.2016.1265633
13. Craig SL, Kourgiantakis T, Kirkland A, Muskat B, Sur D. Riding the wave: pandemic social work in hospitals. *Soc Work Health Care*. 2022;61(5):323–337 PMID: 35786167 doi: 10.1080/00981389.2022.2085232
14. Luther B, Barra J, Martial MA. Essential nursing care management and coordination roles and responsibilities: a content analysis. *Prof Case Manag*. 2019;24(5):249–258 PMID: 31369488 doi: 10.1097/ncm.0000000000000355
15. Alegría M, NeMoyer A, Falgàs Bagué I, Wang Y, Alvarez K. Social determinants of mental health: where we are and where we need to go. *Curr Psychiatry Rep*. 2018;20(11):95 PMID: 30221308 doi: 10.1007/s11920-018-0969-9
16. Fiori KP, Rehm CD, Sanderson D, et al. Integrating social needs screening and community health workers in primary care: the community linkage to care program. *Clin Pediatr (Phila)*. 2020;59(6):547–556 PMID: 32131620 doi: 10.1177/0009922820908589
17. Raphael JL, Rueda A, Lion KC, Giordano TP. The role of lay health workers in pediatric chronic disease: a systematic review. *Acad Pediatr*. 2013;13(5):408–420 PMID: 24011745 doi: 10.1016/j.acap.2013.04.015
18. Murphy JS, Lawton EM, Sandel M. Legal care as part of health care: the benefits of medical-legal partnership. *Pediatr Clin North Am*. 2015;62(5):1263–1271 PMID: 26318951 doi: 10.1016/j.pcl.2015.06.001
19. Bell ON, Hole MK, Johnson K, Marcil LE, Solomon BS, Schickedanz A. Medical-financial partnerships: cross-sector collaborations between medical and financial services to improve health. *Acad Pediatr*. 2020;20(2):166–174 PMID: 31618676 doi: 10.1016/j.acap.2019.10.001
20. *Creating Effective Hospital-Community Partnerships to Build a Culture of Health*. Health Research & Educational Trust; 2016
21. Black S, Sisco S, Williams T, et al. Return on investment from co-locating tax assistance for low-income persons at clinical sites. *JAMA*. 2020;323(11):1093–1095 PMID: 32181840 doi: 10.1001/jama.2020.0545
22. George DR, Rovniak LS, Kraschnewski JL, Morrison KJ, Dillon JF, Bates BY. Medical center farmers markets: a strategic partner in the patient-centered medical home. *Prev Chronic Dis*. 2013;10:E127 PMID: 23906327 doi: 10.5888/pcd10.130105
23. Conti G, Heckman J, Pinto R. The effects of two influential early childhood interventions on health and healthy behaviour. *Econ J (London)*. 2016;126(596):F28–F65 PMID: 28260805 doi: 10.1111/ecoj.12420
24. Daniels D, Wolter-Warmerdam K, Holland S, Hickey F. Reach Out and Read implementation in a pediatric Down syndrome clinic. *J Pediatr Health Care*. 2022;36(3):231–239 PMID: 34879985 doi: 10.1016/j.pedhc.2021.10.003
25. North S, Dooley DG. School-based health care. *Prim Care*. 2020;47(2):231–240 PMID: 32423711 doi: 10.1016/j.pop.2020.02.003
26. Chisholm H, Kershaw T, Sotelo Guerra L, Bocek K, Garcia Y, Lion KC. A realist evaluation analysis of a novel multi-faceted inpatient patient navigation program. *Acad Pediatr*. 2022;22(5):789–796 PMID: 34551342 doi: 10.1016/j.acap.2021.09.009

27. Vais S, Thomson L, Williams A, Sobota A. Rethinking rideshares: a transportation assistance pilot for pediatric patients with sickle cell disease. *J Health Care Poor Underserved.* 2020;31(3):1457–1470 PMID: 33416705 doi: 10.1353/hpu.2020.0105

28. Strane D, Flaherty C, Kellom K, Kenyon CC, Bryant-Stephens T. A health system–initiated intervention to remediate homes of children with asthma. *Pediatrics.* 2023;151(5):e2022058351 PMID: 37042200 doi: 10.1542/peds.2022-058351

29. Bryant-Stephens TC, Strane D, Robinson EK, Bhambhani S, Kenyon CC. Housing and asthma disparities. *J Allergy Clin Immunol.* 2021;148(5):1121–1129 PMID: 34599980 doi: 10.1016/j.jaci.2021.09.023

30. Nofi CP, Roberts BK, Cornell E, et al. Hospital-based violence intervention programs to reduce firearm injuries in children: a scoping review. *J Pediatr Surg.* 2023;58(11):2212–2221 PMID: 37217364 doi: 10.1016/j.jpedsurg.2023.04.020

31. Junior JA, Ha YP, Ruxin TR, et al. A national voter registration campaign. *Pediatrics.* 2023;152(2):e2022059501 PMID: 37465910 doi: 10.1542/peds.2022-059501

Part 3. Future Directions

CHAPTER 9

Medical Trainee Education Around Health-Related Social Needs

Rachel Stein Berman, MD, MPH, FAAP, and Iman Hassan, MD, MS

In this chapter, we describe several frameworks for social determinants of health (SDOH) in medical education and specific strategies for teaching around the SDOH, with a focus on interdisciplinary training to engage with health-related social needs in the clinical setting. We include a model workflow for screening for social needs and placing referrals, discuss documentation of social needs and the plan to address them, describe strategies for communicating with patients about social needs in a trauma-informed and culturally humble way, and share cases that can be used for case-based learning. We discuss how clinical teams can make a bigger impact on addressing SDOH through research, performance improvement, and advocacy projects. Last, we describe methods to evaluate learners engaged in SDOH curricula and discuss future steps to advance medical training in this field.

CHAPTER 9

Medical Trainee Education Around Health-Related Social Needs

Rachel Stein Berman, MD, MPH, FAAP, and Iman Hassan, MD, MS

Introduction

There is growing acknowledgment of the importance of training around the social determinants of health (SDOH) within the health professions and allied fields. Social determinants of health, the conditions in which people are born grow, live, work, and age and the circumstances that shape them, are the greatest predictors of health outcomes and a key contributor to health disparities.[1] Social needs such as transportation needs, housing instability, and food insecurity are downstream manifestations of structural determinants of health most amenable to intervention at the point of clinical care.[2] Interprofessional teamwork to address social needs yields better outcomes for patients.[3] Interdisciplinary medical education training is vital to action on the SDOH. Recognizing that, medical accreditation organizations, such as the Accreditation Council for Graduate Medical Education (ACGME), have called on all specialties to include teaching on SDOH to reduce health disparities.[4] The Association of American Medical Colleges recently released diversity, equity, and inclusion competencies along the learning continuum that incorporate addressing SDOH to promote health equity.[5] In nursing, The National League for Nursing Commission for Nursing Education Accreditation has now incorporated requirements for providing education in the SDOH, health equity, and population health.[6] Social work education has long incorporated assessing, understanding, intervening in, and evaluating the context of the life of an individual, their family, and their community as part of the "person-in-environment" approach. Additionally, social work education highlights the impact of structural forces such as racism, oppression, and systems of power.[7]

Interdisciplinary Teaching of Social Determinants of Health

Key Concept

Teaching clinical teams about SDOH is most effective when all members of an interdisciplinary team are involved in curriculum development and facilitate or participate in teaching sessions. Each team member has valuable expertise to share.

Given that addressing SDOH requires an interdisciplinary approach, teaching clinical teams about SDOH is most effective when all members of an interdisciplinary team are involved. Social workers, community health workers (CHWs), health educators, nurses, nutritionists, physicians, patient advocates or representatives, and other key members of the clinical team should be engaged in curriculum development, reviewing content, and facilitating or participating in teaching sessions.

Training on SDOH must emphasize that every member of the clinical team plays an important role in screening for social needs and in connecting patients to resources. A fundamental principle is that every team member must find their place, acknowledging that other members of the team have different expertise and may be better equipped to work with patients on certain issues. Accordingly, team members need to have clearly defined roles and establish positive working relationships. Furthermore, the workflow for screening and placing referrals for social needs should fit into the clinic's culture and should reflect the different roles and skills of team members.

Clinician and nonclinician champions for social needs screening and referrals who are on the team should be identified and can facilitate the definition of roles, the development and implementation of the workflow, and the design and delivery of SDOH educational sessions for the entire team. Team meetings may be an optimal time to teach about SDOH, to share local and national data and patient stories to motivate screening and referrals, and to obtain feedback on the workflow. Furthermore, clinician and nonclinician champions can meet in smaller working groups to learn from each other's experiences, review individual clinic or institutional data, and share research and policy updates related to SDOH.

There are a growing number of successful examples of interdisciplinary teaching on SDOH in the clinical setting. Community health workers can be invited to attend teaching sessions on SDOH, during which clinicians present the case of a patient with social needs to the CHW, suggest a plan, and obtain feedback on that plan directly from the CHW. Additionally, social workers can play an important role in trainee education on SDOH and patient care. In one curriculum, joint teaching sessions on SDOH were held for medical and physician assistant students during which social work students taught patient engagement strategies. Social workers have also participated in case-based sessions for medical students as part of a longitudinal curriculum on biopsychosocial needs of families and social work perspectives in patient care. These curricula highlight that social workers are a critical asset in patient care, promote interprofessional teaching, and encourage the development of interdisciplinary teamwork skills early on in medical training.[8,9] Furthermore, community partners can play an active role in SDOH education by mentoring trainees, participating in journal clubs and reflective sessions, and facilitating trainee participation in service-learning and community engagement.[10]

Organizational Frameworks for Teaching About Social Determinants of Health

Key Concept

Three core pillars should inform SDOH training program development: education, community, and organization. Principles of trauma-informed care, cultural humility and safety, structural competency, critical consciousness, and systems and design thinking can inform development of SDOH teaching.

In 2016, the National Academies of Sciences, Engineering, and Medicine (NASEM) released *A Framework for Educating Health Professionals to Address the Social Determinants of Health*[11] (**Figure 9-1**). The framework highlights 3 core pillars: education, community, and organization. Education in SDOH should be experiential, integrated, and collaborative, spanning the entire

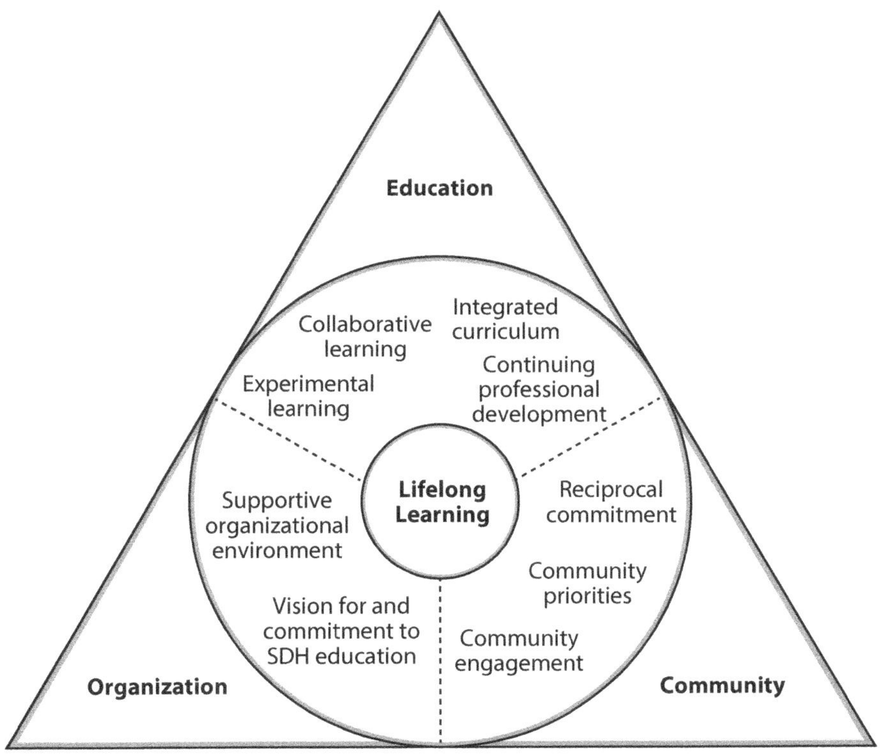

Figure 9-1. National Academies of Sciences, Engineering, and Medicine Framework for Educating Professionals About the Social Determinants of Health

SDH indicates social determinants of health.

Reproduced with permission from Institute of Medicine. *A Framework for Educating Health Professionals to Address the Social Determinants of Health.* National Academies of Sciences, Engineering, and Medicine; 2016. Accessed October 4, 2024. https://www.ncbi.nlm.nih.gov/books/NBK395983.

professional learning continuum. It should incorporate understanding of social, political, and economic factors that affect the health of individuals and populations as well as action on SDOH in the clinical setting. NASEM highlights the essential role that communities play in developing strategies for the creation of learning opportunities that advance health equity. This entails a shifting of power from health professionals to community members and an active prioritization of education based on community needs and building on community assets. Finally, health care organizations are vital in supporting education in SDOH, including commitment to addressing the SDOH and creating an environment that promotes action on SDOH. Additional frameworks have been developed that further expand and conceptualize the education pillar of NASEM's framework. These include trauma-informed care, cultural humility and safety, structural competency, critical consciousness, and systems and design thinking.

Social Needs Through a Trauma-Informed Lens

One framework through which it is important to view and teach SDOH is that of trauma-informed care. Social needs, structural forces, and trauma exist in a cyclical relationship. Larger traumatic structural forces, including racism, police brutality, war, and economic policies, cause people to have social needs, and having social needs itself is a form of trauma. Social needs thus need to be framed not as an individual's fault but as the result of structural forces, which also contribute to an individual's experience of trauma in the form of community violence, domestic violence, and crime.

Viewing SDOH through a trauma-informed lens encourages a strengths-based approach to addressing social needs. Trauma-informed care shifts the perspective from "What is wrong with you?" to "What has happened to you?" removing blame and promoting a more compassionate approach that allows for healing.[12] Trauma-informed care emphasizes empowerment, ensuring that individuals are heard and are given the opportunity to make decisions for themselves.[13] Furthermore, trauma-informed care focuses on resilience, promoting individuals' strengths and assets.[14]

Trauma-informed care also necessitates the practice of cultural humility and establishes equity as a gold standard. Viewing SDOH through the lens of trauma-informed care requires recognition of current and past structural violence and structural racism, the trauma they have caused, and the need to collectively oppose these structural forces to advance equity and address social needs.[15]

Through its strengths-based and culturally humble approach, addressing SDOH in a trauma-informed way reduces the unintended consequences of screening for social needs. Although such screening has clear benefits, it may also have inadvertent harms.[16] Questions about SDOH are sensitive. These questions may make patients feel vulnerable, and physicians asking these questions may feel uncomfortable and concerned that they will lose their patients' trust. Additionally, addressing social determinants in diverse patient populations requires interdisciplinary teamwork and robust care coordination that are difficult to attain. Screening without the ability to provide appropriate treatment and referrals has been considered ineffective and unethical. Teaching teams to address SDOH in a trauma-informed way can mitigate these potential unintended harms.

Cultural Humility and Safety

Social determinants of health need to be understood and taught to clinical teams through a framework of cultural humility and cultural safety. As noted in the Social Needs Through a Trauma-Informed Lens section earlier in this chapter, practicing cultural humility is one aspect of trauma-informed care, and it is also a step toward achieving the ideal of cultural safety. According to the First Nations Health Authority, "[c]ultural humility is a process of self-reflection to understand personal and systemic biases and to develop and maintain respectful processes and relationships based on mutual trust. Cultural humility involves humbly acknowledging oneself as a learner when it comes to understanding another's experience." The end goal of this process is cultural safety, which the First Nations Health Authority defines as "an outcome based on respectful engagement that recognizes and strives to address power imbalances inherent in the health care system. It results in an environment free of racism and discrimination, where people feel safe when receiving health care."[17] Establishing an environment of cultural safety through the ongoing process of practicing cultural humility is critical to providing structurally competent and trauma-informed care, both of which are essential to address SDOH.

Structural Competency

Structural competency was developed in 2014 by Drs Jonathan Metzl and Helena Hansen. It has 5 major principles: (1) recognizing the upstream social, economic, and political structures that shape behavior, illness, and health; (2) developing an "extra-clinical" language of structure that draws on fields such as anthropology, urban planning, and economics; (3) recognizing the structural forces that mediate "cultural" barriers; (4) observing and imagining structural interventions; and (5) developing structural humility by acknowledging the complexity of structures and recognizing the limits of medical expertise.[18] Structural competency has been used to develop a number of curricula, toolkits, and teaching scenarios that we explore in the Resources section later in this chapter.

Critical Consciousness

Critical consciousness, derived from the work of educator Paulo Freire, and critical theory, developed by the Frankfurt School, involve a reflective awareness of differences in power, privilege, and inequities within social relationships and a reorientation toward social justice.[19] To do this, education needs to move beyond models that transfer knowledge from teacher to learner (thereby maintaining the status quo) and instead connect learners with their own personal, cognitive, and emotional experience; promote engagement in dialogue; challenge dominant narratives; and emancipate learners and others through collaborative problem-solving and action. A 2017 review of health professions education that fosters critical consciousness revealed several key components of this type of pedagogy: incorporating personal experience; appreciating context, including communities, systems, and broader relationships; illuminating power structures, including those present in education and health care; providing space for critical reflection; and promoting equity and social justice within communities. Incorporating these components allows learners to recognize the social and political nature of education and health care, grapple with the influences of power and privilege on care delivery, and examine assumptions that further existing systems of oppression. The authors offer several specific practices to foster critical consciousness, which include promoting authentic dialogue, recognizing the value of everyone in the room, sharing and inviting stories, questioning the status quo, creating cognitive disequilibrium, and challenging the power hierarchy.[20]

Systems Thinking and Design Thinking

Systems thinking is a holistic approach to transforming complex social systems such as health care education or delivery. It involves understanding how elements of a system interact with each other over time and what the root causes of systems defects are and involves acting on "high-leverage areas" that result in system redesign. Like systems thinking, design thinking is an outcomes-focused approach that entails understanding the needs of the end user (learner and teacher centeredness), using collective brainstorming to produce creative solutions, engaging in prototyping and experimentation, and making timely adjustments based on feedback from potential users.[21] Dr Jed Gonzalo and others have incorporated systems thinking into their conceptual model for health systems science (HSS), which attempts to elucidate the ACGME systems-based practice competency along a continuum that encompasses both undergraduate and graduate medical education. Part of HSS is the concept of physicians as "systems citizens," whose professional identity formation is centered not simply on their biomedical acumen but on their role in coproducing health care delivery transformation with patients and communities to achieve ideal patient outcomes.[22]

Social Determinants of Health Education Within the Clinical Practice Environment

Key Concept

Training on SDOH for clinical teams should include the following:

- The importance of expanding or rethinking the traditional social history
- The social needs screening tools available for use in the clinical setting
- The clinical workflow for screening for social needs and making appropriate referrals
- Community resources available
- How to appropriately document social needs and the plan to address them, including follow-up
- Communication strategies for discussing social needs with patients that are trauma informed and culturally humble.

Reimagining the Social History

The increasing recognition of the impact of social circumstances on health outcomes has necessitated an expansion of the social history elicited during clinical encounters. Traditionally, a pediatric social history includes where and with whom a patient lives, whether they have pets, whether anyone at home smokes, and what the child aspires to be when they grow up. The expanded social history also includes access to food, housing quality and stability, access to transportation and health care, perception of health care and relevant previous experiences, neighborhood safety and safety at home, experiences of trauma and racism, immigration status and need for legal assistance, family structure, spiritual beliefs, and health literacy, among others.[23,24] It is important to acknowledge that not all items can be discussed in a single visit, and it is often more prudent to explore certain social triggers of the patient's manifesting symptoms or chief concern. Furthermore, the patient's neighborhood characteristics can be considered through measures such as the Social Vulnerability Index, which uses US Census variables to identify communities that may need more support, specifically in natural and human-caused disasters.[25]

Social Needs Screening

Beyond eliciting an expanded social history, universal screening for SDOH is now recommended by the American Academy of Pediatrics (AAP).[26] Many screening tools are available for use in the clinical setting,[27] and the screening tool that is chosen should be reviewed with the entire team. Embedding the screening tool into the electronic health record (EHR) facilitates a team's ability to address patients' social needs, as it enables all team members to upload responses after screening and to review responses before placing referrals and sharing appropriate resources.

Workflow for Screening and Referrals

During an educational session, the clinic workflow for screening for social needs and making appropriate referrals should also be reviewed, and the team should provide feedback, particularly on how the workflow fits into the culture of the clinic (**Figure 9-2**). Team members should

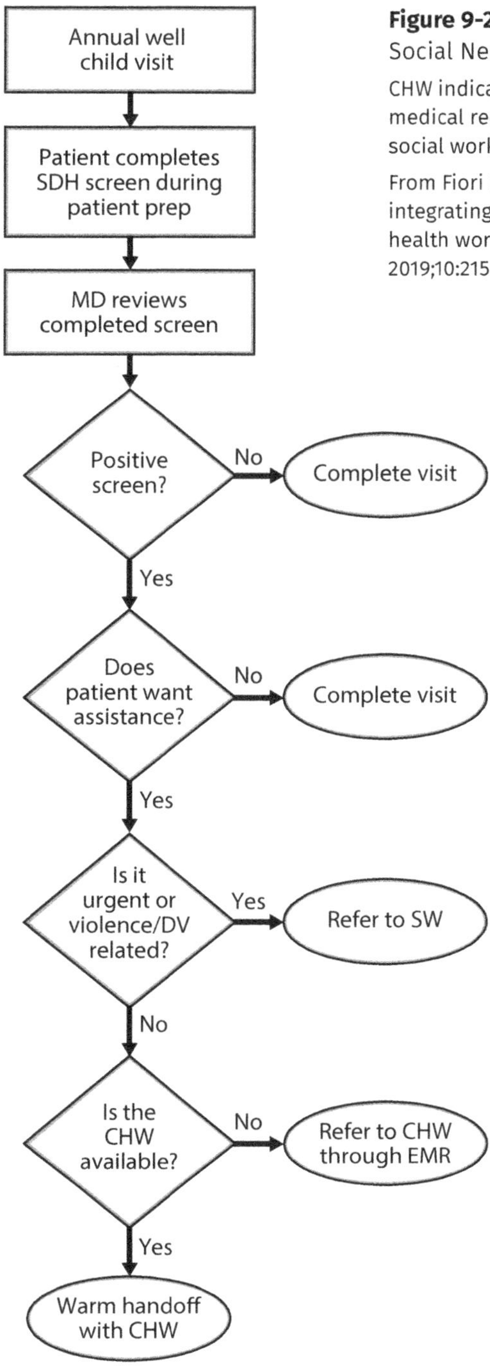

Figure 9-2. Community Linkage to Care Health Center Workflow for Social Needs Screening and Community Health Worker Referrals

CHW indicates community health worker; DV, domestic violence; EMR, electronic medical record; MD, medical doctor; SDH, social determinants of health; and SW, social worker.

From Fiori K, Patel M, Sanderson D, et al. From policy statement to practice: integrating social needs screening and referral assistance with community health workers in urban academic health center. *J Prim Care Comm Health.* 2019;10:2150132719899207.

be provided with information about resources to address social needs. Although their role in the workflow may not be to share resources directly with patients, team members should be aware of the resources that exist and may share these resources directly if a patient declines a referral to another team member or if that team member is unavailable. Team members should also understand that it is critical to follow up with patients about their social needs and whether they succeeded in connecting to resources. This follow-up should be part of the workflow.

Communication Strategies

How we communicate with patients about social needs is as important as how we elicit their social needs. Frameworks for training around social needs communication should be trauma informed[28] and relationship centered[29] and maintain a strengths-based approach.[30] These approaches can work synergistically to guide specific social needs communication skills in ways that avoid stigma and microaggressions. Key components include asking permission from patients, explaining rationale, invoking shared values, starting with open-ended questions, expressing appreciation for patient disclosures, acknowledging hardship, eliciting strengths, prioritizing social needs, eliciting past experiences, and being transparent about information sharing with patients.[29] Educators at the University of Cincinnati developed videotaped vignettes to help train resident physicians in counseling patients around social needs.[31] There are ongoing efforts to develop a validated checklist of social needs communications skills for use in observed, structured clinical encounters and direct observation.

Structural Analysis

Structural analysis is a step-by-step method for incorporating SDOH into clinical reasoning and a framework for operationalizing structural competency in clinical care during ambulatory and inpatient clinical teaching. Structural analysis starts with creating a patient-centered clinical problem list. It explicitly calls for identifying structural and social root causes of clinical problems by using a root-cause analysis approach (**Figure 9-3**) and constructing a prioritized structural problem list that incorporates root causes. Finally, it involves brainstorming solutions to address structural barriers and social needs that center patient's experiences, draw on established relationships within institutions and communities, and maintain a strengths-based approach.[32]

Documentation of structural and social barriers in the health record can help reduce stigmatizing language by framing clinical narratives around forces and influences that fundamentally affect health and away from isolated personal behaviors that can foster patient blaming.[32] Studies have shown that stigmatizing or biased language in the health record can influence clinical outcomes.[33] Best practices to highlight when training around documentation include avoiding explicit documentation of social needs with potential legal ramifications, such as undocumented status; being transparent with patients about social needs documentation; including individual and community strengths in documentation; and keeping problem lists updated to reflect changing needs and barriers.[32] Care must also be taken to specifically avoid propagating racial and ethnic bias in documentation.[34] Several *International Classification of Diseases, 10th Revision,* codes (specifically Z59 codes) allow for inclusion of social needs in medical problem lists.[35]

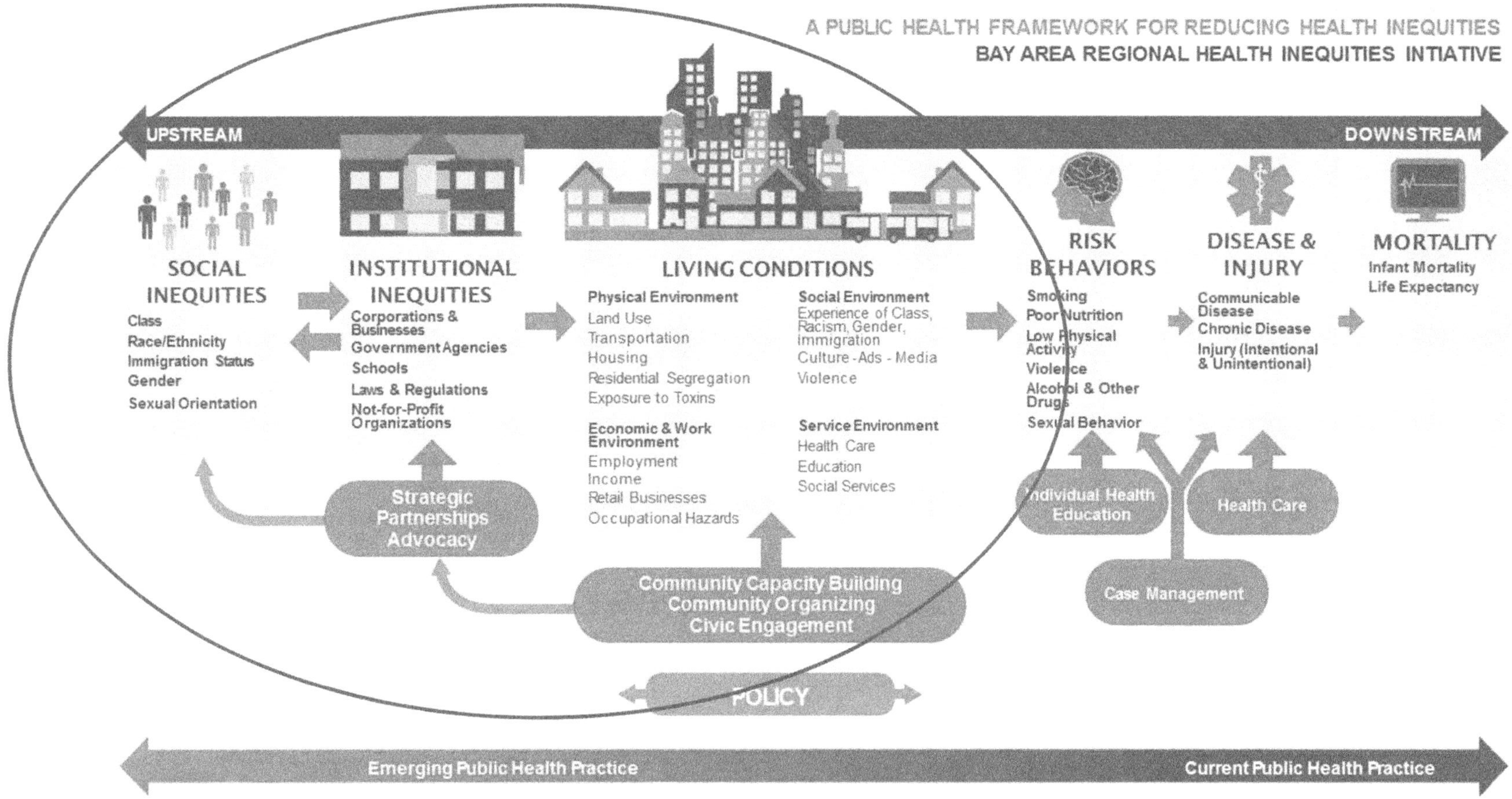

Figure 9-3. Identifying Root Structural Causes of Health Outcomes

Reproduced with permission from Bay Area Regional Health Inequities Initiative. BARHII framework. Accessed May 3, 2024. https://barhii.org/framework.

Teaching Tools/Strategies for Social Determinants of Health in Clinical Practice

Key Concept

Several strategies have been pioneered for teaching SDOH. These include case-based learning, experiential learning through simulations and neighborhood/home visits, and free open-access medical education (FOAM) through online or social media content.

Several strategies for embedding SDOH education into medical education have been published and include guidance on structurally competent clinical teaching cases, experiential learning, and FOAM. For all strategies, both reinforced, spaced-apart learning sessions and active collaboration with interdisciplinary partners and community members should be essential components of curriculum design and development.

Case-based learning can be a powerful tool for illustrating the impact of SDOH on clinical care. Several examples of structurally competent teaching cases have been published, most notably the *New England Journal of Medicine* Case Studies in Social Medicine.[36] Additional examples include the social medicine cases published by the University of Pittsburgh School of Medicine[37] and teaching cases published as part of the Alliance for Academic Internal Medicine Patient Experience subgroup of the Health Disparities Collaborative.[38] Educators at the Albert Einstein College of Medicine in the Bronx, NY, are currently working to develop structurally competent morbidity and mortality conferences and clinical reasoning seminars. In 2019, Krishnan and colleagues published a guide for revising clinical teaching cases to incorporate structural competency. They highlighted the need to treat race as a social construct rather than a biological construct and avoid listing race as a "risk factor" for disease or pathologizing race; to explicitly include structural and social contributors, such as racism, as part of case histories; to avoid reductionist portrayals of cultures other than North American and Western European; and to include a diverse range of patient and clinician portrayals and images.[39]

Experiential learning, developed by David Kolb, provides the added benefit over case-based learning of offering learners the opportunity to learn by performing skills and reflecting on their experience.[40] One example of the use of experiential learning to teach SDOH is the incorporation of simulations to sensitize learners to structural and social barriers that patients or others may face while experiencing poverty.[41,42] Privilege walks have been used to foster reflection on the interplay between privilege, power, and SDOH.[43] Buitron de la Vega and coworkers at Boston Medical Center have pioneered the use of virtual reality–simulated learning environments to engage learners in interprofessional SDOH training.[8] Observed structural clinical encounters and unannounced standardized patients can be powerful experiential teaching methods for training on communication skills needed to address SDOH in clinical encounters with patients.[44] Finally, the use of neighborhood and patient home visits to teach about SDOH has been shown to improve knowledge, attitudes, and behaviors.[45]

Increasingly, FOAM through videos, social media posts, podcasts, and "Tweetorials" have helped shed light on SDOH and disseminate anti-racist medical education practices. Notable examples are the *Antiracism in Medicine* podcast by the Clinical Problem Solvers[46] and the *Social*

Interventions Research & Evaluation Network (SIREN) podcast.[47] A growing number of medical education journals have also released podcasts that tackle SDOH, including *Health Affairs*.[48] At the Montefiore Health System, SDOH Tweetorials were shown to improve resident physician knowledge and competency.[49]

Teaching on Specific Social Determinants of Health

As noted in the Teaching Tools/Strategies for Social Determinants of Health in Clinical Practice section earlier in this chapter, case-based learning, long-recognized as an effective teaching method in medical education,[50] can be used to teach about specific SDOH, such as housing quality and food security. Key components of case-based learning for specific SDOH include sharing background data at the local, state, national, and international levels; identifying social and structural factors contributing to the patient's presentation and including these factors in documentation; and developing a plan that addresses the patient's social needs by connecting them to appropriate resources that aim to overcome structural barriers. Here are 2 examples of cases that can be shared with clinical teams to teach on specific SDOH.

Example 1

An 8-year-old girl has an appointment with her pediatrician to follow up about her asthma. She had been in the emergency department 3 times in the previous 2 weeks for cough and difficulty breathing. At each visit, she was given nebulized albuterol and ipratropium, her symptoms improved, and she was discharged home. She was also treated with oral corticosteroids and azithromycin. Her mother reports that she is taking her inhaled medications, oral corticosteroids, and antibiotic as directed, but her symptoms have persisted. On further history taking, her mother reports that she herself, the patient, and the patient's younger brother are living in a shelter. They had moved 3 times in the past month because their shelter apartment had no heat or hot water. The patient's mother tried using the stove to heat the apartment, but it had a strange odor, so she turned it off, concerned that it would make the patient's asthma worse. The patient missed 8 days of school during this period.

Background Data From 2022

United States: 582,462 people experienced homelessness, 28% of which were families with children.

- New York State: 74,178 people experienced homelessness. State of homelessness: 2023 edition. National Alliance to End Homelessness. Accessed May 6, 2024. https://endhomelessness.org/homelessness-in-america/homelessness-statistics/state-of-homelessness/#homelessness-in-2022.
- New York City: 28.3% of households reported severe rent burden, 9,800 families with children were living in shelters, more than 20% of housing units filed maintenance complaints in lower-income neighborhoods, including the Bronx.
- Bronx, NY: 33.6% of households reported severe rent burden. *Keeping Track of New York City's Children: 2022*. Citizens' Committee for Children of New York; 2022. Accessed May 3, 2024. https://data.cccnewyork.org.

Assessment and Plan

This patient has severe persistent asthma with several recent asthma exacerbations. Her home environment, specifically housing instability and resulting poor housing quality (including lack of heat), and a possible smoke inhalation exposure are known triggers for asthma exacerbations. Her severe asthma has resulted in missed school days, which are known to affect learning outcomes. In addition to ensuring this patient has access to her maintenance inhalers and education on inhaler techniques, it is important for the clinician to inquire about and provide resources for housing and education on housing to this patient and her family.

- Housing instability and poor housing conditions exacerbating asthma
  - Refer this patient to a home asthma program that can inspect the patient's current housing for asthma triggers. Home asthma programs work with a team of social workers and lawyers to quickly resolve poor housing conditions and even to treat triggers such as mold and rodents. Referral to a medical-legal partnership may also be helpful if there are delays in fixing housing conditions.
  - Provide a physician's letter advocating for this patient to be placed into permanent housing more quickly in response to her underlying severe asthma and risk for additional complications, including more asthma exacerbations, intubation, and death, without a safe and stable home.
  - Screen this patient and her family for other social needs, such as transportation services (often patients within the shelter system can be relocated to areas far from their medical home), medication affordability, and food insecurity (financial insecurity, which leads to inability to pay rent, can also lead to inability to afford food, medications, and other essential items).
- Missed school days
  - Provide a letter to this patient's school administrators explaining her absences from school and requesting assistance for the patient to catch up with learning and schoolwork.
  - Provide an asthma medication administration form that enables the school nurse to give inhaled asthma medications at school as needed.
  - Provide an asthma action plan for the parent and school.

Example 2

An 8-month-old boy presents to the pediatrician for a health supervision visit. He has not been to the clinic since 2 months of age (he missed the 4- and 6-month visits). His mother reports that he is feeding well, taking 5 oz of formula 5 times a day as well as taking pureed foods 3 times a day. His weight was noted to be less than the 3rd percentile (down from the 18th percentile), and his height was following the curve at the 15th percentile. He is meeting his developmental milestones. On further history taking, his mother reports that she has been mixing the baby's formula with 2 scoops for each 5 oz of water, which is diluting the baby's formula, because she was running out and did not have money to buy more formula.

Background Data From 2022

- United States: 17.3% of households with children (6.4 million households) and 7.3 million children in the United States were experiencing food insecurity or were uncertain of having or unable to obtain enough food. Food security status of US households with children in 2022. USDA Economic Research Service. Accessed October 7, 2024. https://www.ers.usda.gov/topics/food-nutrition-assistance/food-security-in-the-u-s/key-statistics-graphics/#children.
- New York City: 15% of households with children reported food insufficiency (sometimes or often not having enough food to eat). *Keeping Track of New York City's Children: 2022.* Citizens' Committee for Children of New York; 2022. Accessed October 7, 2024. https://data.cccnewyork.org.

- Bronx, NY: 36% of residents were experiencing food insecurity. Chatterjee D, Hinojosa J. *The Big Apple's Bitter Bite: Food Hardship in New York City.* Community Service Society; 2023. Accessed October 7, 2024. https://smhttp-ssl-58547.nexcesscdn.net/nycss/images/uploads/pubs/Food_Insecurity_V41.pdf.

Assessment and Plan

This patient has severe underweight caused by food insecurity. Low weight has been shown to result in increased risk for infection, developmental delay, and long-term health conditions. Addressing this family's food insecurity is critical.

- Food insecurity resulting in low weight
  - Refer this patient and his family to programs that distribute free formula to prevent the mother from having to dilute formula supplies.
  - Complete the provider form for the Special Supplemental Nutrition Program for Women, Infants, and Children (WIC) and refer the mother to a WIC enrollment center. WIC provides money for essential items such as formula.
  - Inquire about interest in other food assistance programs to help family members affected by food insecurity, such as food banks, soup kitchens, and the Supplemental Nutrition Assistance Program, which provides money for food. Food insecurity usually affects entire families, and these assistance programs can help.

Screen this patient and his family for other social needs, such as financial insecurity and rent and utility arrears. This patient may benefit from assistance for these other social needs, which can co-occur with food insecurity.

Team Projects to Improve Social Determinants of Health: Moving Upstream

Key Concept

In addition to educational sessions on SDOH, clinical teams can further their learning and commitment to addressing SDOH through research, performance improvement, and advocacy projects.

Beyond educational sessions on SDOH, teams can further grow their expertise and share their work through research, performance improvement, and advocacy projects. These projects, like the educational sessions, will be most effective when members of an interdisciplinary team are involved.

Many examples of qualitative and quantitative research projects on screening and referring for social needs can be found in the literature. These studies may be descriptive, in which multiple clinics within the same institution or across institutions collaborate to collect and share data on the number of patients screened, which social needs were positive, and whether and how these needs were addressed.[51,52] These studies may also be randomized controlled trials, during which an intervention to address social needs is assessed for feasibility, efficacy, and/or cost effectiveness.[53] SIREN is an excellent resource for research on SDOH.[47]

Smaller-scale performance improvement projects are critical as well. Clinical teams should be encouraged to implement screening and referring for social needs in different iterations, each slightly improved from the first to increase the number of patients screened and referred. In these iterations, or Plan-Do-Study-Act cycles, teams seek to address SDOH most efficiently and equitably. Different iterations of the workflow may include adding the social needs screening tool to an existing packet of screening tools given to patients when they arrive in clinic, placing stickers on computer screens to remind clinicians to upload paper screening tools into the EHR, and flagging positive screening results in the EHR to remind clinicians to refer to a CHW or social worker if the patient accepts. For example, a pediatric hematology clinic used quality improvement methods to optimize the process of screening for social needs and making referrals to local resources.[54]

We cannot optimally address SDOH without looking further upstream at the policies, systems, and other structural forces that lead to social needs and inequities. Team members can work together to influence policymakers and to encourage patients to be civically engaged. There is a growing interest in civic health, and civic participation is now considered an SDOH for Healthy People 2030.[55] Vot-ER is an advocacy group that is leading the way in increasing voter registration and encouraging voter participation in the health care setting.[56] Additionally, many professional groups, including the AAP, have advocacy campaigns for clinicians to voice the needs of children who cannot vote themselves. For example, when the New York State legislature was negotiating the state budget in the spring of 2023, pediatricians were encouraged to call and email their elected officials to promote inclusion of universal free school meals, continuous Medicaid coverage for children 0 to 6 years old, and a working families tax credit within the budget. Pediatricians were given information about each of these items and were directed to their legislators' contact information. (AAP New York Chapter 3, email to Dr Berman, April 17, 2023). Furthermore, for clinical teams interested in local advocacy projects, the AAP Community Pediatrics Training Initiative (CPTI) contains a toolkit to facilitate the implementation of child health advocacy projects. The CPTI toolkit has been used by different institutions to develop advocacy training curricula for students and residents, to provide professional development for practicing physicians, and to provide guidance for the implementation of community-based interventions.[57]

Evaluation of Learners

Key Concept

Social determinants of health learner assessments with reliability and validity evidence are still under development, but behavioral checklists, observed standardized clinical encounters, case-based application, qualitative reflection, and clinical behavioral metrics show promise in SDOH training evaluation.

A national survey of US medical schools and physician assistant programs conducted in 2020 revealed a wide variation in how training programs evaluate education in SDOH. Most programs responding reported assessing learner knowledge, attitudes, and skills with less than half of programs incorporating a behavioral assessment. Medical schools were more likely to assess interpersonal and communication skills, patient care, and systems-based practice, while physician assistant schools were more likely to assess society and population health, health literacy and communication, and patient-centered practice knowledge. Locally developed tools without formal validity evidence were the most common sources of assessment. Respondents reported that lack of agreement on what "SDOH competency" meant and lack of faculty training in SDOH assessment were major barriers.[58]

A small number of formal assessment tools are starting to emerge. In 2021, Hsia and coworkers developed a structural competency instrument to assess a longitudinal health equity curriculum for pharmacy students.[59] There is ongoing multi-institutional work by faculty at the Albert Einstein College of Medicine, University of Pittsburgh School of Medicine, Columbia University Vagelos School of Physicians and Surgeons, and Dell Seton Medical Center at the University of Texas at Austin to develop and validate a simplified structural competency assessment tool. The Critical Consciousness Scale has also been validated in a general population and may have useful applications in medical education assessment.[60] There are also a number of health care disparities assessments that incorporate cultural sensitivity and humility.[61]

Given the complex, multifaceted nature of SDOH, stand-alone surveys are likely to be insufficient to evaluate training programs and clinic-based SDOH education. Multi-model assessments using observed standardized clinical encounters, case-based application, qualitative reflection, and clinical behavioral metrics are more likely to provide useful, holistic evaluation. Clinical behavioral assessments may include direct observation; unannounced standardized patients; and monitoring of clinical dashboards for rates of social needs screening, documentation practices around SDOH, and rates of referrals to interdisciplinary and community partners.

Conclusion

With the awareness that social and environmental factors determine 80% to 90% of our health outcomes,[1] teaching health profession students, residents, and clinical teams about SDOH and how to practically screen for and address social needs is essential. Addressing social needs requires an interdisciplinary approach, as team members have unique skills and expertise to work with patients on different issues. Social determinants of health education for clinical teams must therefore be interdisciplinary, such that all team members are engaged in developing curriculum and in facilitating or participating in teaching sessions.

Several frameworks can guide teaching about SDOH using a strengths-based, structural approach. Social determinants of health training should be informed by 3 pillars: education, community, and engagement. Additional frameworks that expand on the pillars of education include those of trauma-informed care, cultural humility and safety, structural competency, critical consciousness, and systems and design thinking. These frameworks inform the content of educational sessions, teaching strategies, and the evaluation of learners.

Next steps for SDOH education are to develop more evidence-based tools for the professional development of clinical teams so they can address social needs and more evidence-based strategies for the evaluation of curricula and learners. More robust training will in turn inspire practice improvement and advocacy, from the level of the individual patient to that of our complex health care system.

Resources

- Academic Pediatric Association US Child Poverty Curriculum: www.aap.org/en/patient-care/poverty-and-child-health/academic-pediatric-association-us-child-poverty-curriculum
- American Academy of Family Physicians Health Equity Curricular Toolkit and The EveryONE Project: www.aafp.org/family-physician/patient-care/the-everyone-project/health-equity-tools.html and www.aafp.org/family-physician/patient-care/the-everyone-project.html
- American Academy of Pediatrics Community Pediatrics Training Initiative advocacy toolkit: www.aap.org/en/advocacy/community-health-and-advocacy/teach-community-health-and-advocacy
- American College of Chest Physicians Caring with Compassion: https://caringwithcompassion.org/educators
- Center for Community Health and Development at the University of Kansas Community toolbox: https://ctb.ku.edu/en/table-of-contents/analyze/analyze-community-problems-and-solutions/social-determinants-of-health/main
- Centers for Disease Control and Prevention *Health and Well-Being for All* meeting-in-a-box: www.cdcfoundation.org/health-in-a-box
- Greater New York Hospital Association social determinants of health in primary care residency training: www.gnyha.org/tool/training-primary-care-residents-on-the-social-determinants-of-health
- Health Disparities Collaborative of the Alliance for Academic Internal Medicine: www.im.org/resources/ume-gme-program-resources/resources-disparities
- *MedEdPORTAL* anti-racism publications: www.mededportal.org/anti-racism
- National Collaboration for Education to Address the Social Determinants of Health database of curricula: https://sdoheducation.org
- Robert Wood Johnson Foundation *A New Way to Talk About Social Determinants of Health*: www.health.state.mn.us/communities/practice/resources/equitylibrary/rwjf-newwaytotalk.html
- Unnatural Causes: https://unnaturalcauses.org/for_educators.php

Key Points

- Education in the SDOH is now part of accreditation guidelines for all health care professionals.
- Addressing SDOH requires an interdisciplinary approach; teaching clinical teams about SDOH is most effective when all members of an interdisciplinary team are involved.
- Several frameworks can guide teaching about SDOH with a strengths-based, structural approach. These frameworks include those of trauma-informed care, cultural humility and safety, structural competency, critical consciousness, and systems and design thinking. These frameworks inform the content of educational sessions, teaching strategies, and the evaluation of learners.
- Key components for incorporating SDOH into clinical practice include reimagining the social history, incorporating social needs screening and associated clinical workflows, training on communication strategies, and fostering structural analysis.
- Next steps for SDOH education are to develop more evidence-based tools for the professional development of clinical teams so they can address social needs and more evidence-based strategies for the evaluation of curricula and learners.

References

1. Hood CM, Gennuso KP, Swain GR, Catlin BB. County health rankings: relationships between determinant factors and health outcomes. *Am J Prev Med.* 2016;50(2):129–135 PMID: 26526164 doi: 10.1016/j.amepre.2015.08.024
2. Alderwick H, Gottlieb LM. Meanings and misunderstandings: a social determinants of health lexicon for health care systems. *Milbank Q.* 2019;97(2):407–419 PMID: 31069864 doi: 10.1111/1468-0009.12390
3. Cheng I, Powers K, Mange D, et al. Interprofessional education through healthcare hotspotting: understanding social determinants of health and mastering complex care through teamwork. *J Interprof Educ Pract.* 2020;20:1000340 doi: 10.1016/j.xjep.2020.100340
4. Koh NJ, Wagner R, Newton RC, Kuhn CM, Co JPT, Weiss KB; CLER Evaluation Committee, CLER Program. *CLER National Report of Findings.* Accreditation Council for Graduate Medical Education; 2021 doi: 10.35425/ACGME.0008
5. Association of American Medical Colleges. *Diversity, Equity, and Inclusion Competencies Across the Learning Continuum.* Association of American Medical Colleges; 2022. Accessed May 3, 2024. http://resource.nlm.nih.gov/9918504888906676
6. Shellenbarger T. Accreditors stepping up to the challenge: reimagining the future of nursing. *Teach Learn Nurs.* 2022;17(3):253–255 PMID: 35440919 doi: 10.1016/j.teln.2022.03.004
7. Competencies. Boston University School of Social Work. Accessed May 3, 2024. https://www.bu.edu/ssw/academics/msw/competencies
8. Buitron de la Vega P, Dimitri N, Araujo Brinkerhoff C, et al. Virtual reality simulated learning environments: a strategy to teach interprofessional students about social determinants of health. *Acad Med.* 2022;97(12):1799–1803 PMID: 35703204 doi: 10.1097/ACM.0000000000004776
9. Martinez I, Lourdes M, Hayden MH, Balmaceda V. Incorporating social work perspectives into interprofessional health teams: engaging students in a biopsychosocial assessment of family. *MedEdPORTAL.* 2014;10:9915 doi: 10.15766/mep_2374-8265.9915
10. Chung EK, Kahn S, Altshuler M, Lane JL, Plumb J. The JeffSTARS Advocacy and Community Partnership Elective: a closer look at child health advocacy in action. *MedEdPORTAL.* 2016;12:10526 PMID: 30800729 doi: 10.15766/mep_2374-8265.10526
11. Institute of Medicine. *A Framework for Educating Health Professionals to Address the Social Determinants of Health.* National Academies of Sciences, Engineering, and Medicine; 2016
12. Understanding trauma & stress. University of California San Francisco. Accessed May 3, 2024. https://hearts.ucsf.edu/understanding-trauma-stress
13. Empowerment & collaboration. University of California San Francisco. Accessed May 3, 2024. https://hearts.ucsf.edu/empowerment-collaboration
14. Resilience & social-emotional wellness. University of California San Francisco. Accessed May 3, 2024. https://hearts.ucsf.edu/resilience-social-emotional-wellness
15. Cultural humility & equity. University of California San Francisco. Accessed May 3, 2024. https://hearts.ucsf.edu/cultural-humility-equity
16. Garg A, Boynton-Jarrett R, Dworkin PH. Avoiding the unintended consequences of screening for social determinants of health. *JAMA.* 2016;316(8):813–814 PMID: 27367226 doi: 10.1001/jama.2016.9282
17. Cultural safety and humility. First Nations Health Authority. Accessed May 3, 2024. https://www.fnha.ca/what-we-do/cultural-safety-and-humility
18. Metzl JM, Hansen H. Structural competency: theorizing a new medical engagement with stigma and inequality. *Soc Sci Med.* 2014;103:126–133 PMID: 24507917 doi: 10.1016/j.socscimed.2013.06.032

19. Kumagai AK, Lypson ML. Beyond cultural competence: critical consciousness, social justice, and multicultural education. *Acad Med.* 2009;84(6):782–787 PMID: 19474560 doi: 10.1097/ACM.0b013e3181a42398

20. Halman M, Baker L, Ng S. Using critical consciousness to inform health professions education: a literature review. *Perspect Med Educ.* 2017;6(1):12–20 PMID: 28050879 doi: 10.1007/s40037-016-0324-y

21. Hassan IS, AbdulKareem AK, Alrabee NHK, et al. A systems thinking approach for the creation of effective competency-based medical education programs. *Pan Afr Med J.* 2022;41:203 PMID: 35685098 doi: 10.11604/pamj.2022.41.203.28896

22. Gonzalo JD, Chang A, Dekhtyar M, Starr SR, Holmboe E, Wolpaw DR. Health systems science in medical education: unifying the components to catalyze transformation. *Acad Med.* 2020;95(9):1362–1372 PMID: 32287080 doi: 10.1097/ACM.0000000000003400

23. Kenyon C, Sandel M, Silverstein M, Shakir A, Zuckerman B. Revisiting the social history for child health. *Pediatrics.* 2007;120(3):e734–e738 PMID: 17766513 doi: 10.1542/peds.2006-2495

24. Behforouz HL, Drain PK, Rhatigan JJ. Rethinking the social history. *N Engl J Med.* 2014;371(14):1277–1279 PMID: 25271600 doi: 10.1056/NEJMp1404846

25. Agency for Toxic Substances and Disease Registry. CDC/ATSDR Social Vulnerability Index. Centers for Disease Control and Prevention. Accessed May 3, 2024. https://www.atsdr.cdc.gov/placeandhealth/svi/index.html

26. American Academy of Pediatrics Council on Community Pediatrics. Poverty and child health in the United States. *Pediatrics.* 2016;137(4):e20160339 PMID: 26962238 doi: 10.1542/peds.2016-0339

27. Committee on Integrating Social Needs Care Into the Delivery of Health Care. *Integrating Social Needs Care Into the Delivery of Health Care: Moving Upstream to Improve the Nation's Health.* National Academies of Sciences, Engineering, and Medicine; 2019

28. *Screening for Social Needs: Guiding Care Teams to Engage Patients.* American Hospital Association; 2019. Accessed May 3, 2024. https://www.aha.org/toolkitsmethodology/2019-06-05-screening-social-needs-guiding-care-teams-engage-patients

29. Schoenthaler A, Hassan I, Fiscella K. The time is now: fostering relationship-centered discussions about patients' social determinants of health. *Patient Educ Couns.* 2019;102(4):810–814 PMID: 30391299 doi: 10.1016/j.pec.2018.10.025

30. Flacks J, Boynton-Jarrett R. *Strengths-Based Approach to Screening Families for Health-Related Social Needs.* MLPB, Center for the Study of Social Policy; 2018

31. Klein MD, Alcamo AM, Beck AF, et al. Can a video curriculum on the social determinants of health affect residents' practice and families' perceptions of care? *Acad Pediatr.* 2014;14(2):159–166 PMID: 24602579 doi: 10.1016/j.acap.2013.11.002

32. Hassan IF, Bui T. The structural analysis: incorporating structurally competent clinical reasoning into case-based presentations. *J Gen Intern Med.* 2022;37(13):3465–3470 PMID: 35922707 doi: 10.1007/s11606-022-07751-7

33. Goddu AP, O'Conor KJ, Lanzkron S, et al. Do words matter? stigmatizing language and the transmission of bias in the medical record. *J Gen Intern Med.* 2018;33(5):685–691 PMID: 29374357 doi: 10.1007/s11606-017-4289-2

34. Williams JC, Andreou A, Castillo EG, et al. Antiracist documentation practices—shaping clinical encounters and decision making. *N Engl J Med.* 2023;389(13):1238–1244 PMID: 37754291 doi: 10.1056/NEJMms2303340

35. Proposed guidance on utilizing *ICD-10* Z codes for social determinants of health diagnoses. Greater New York Hospital Association, Healthcare Association of New York State, Community Health Center Association of New York State, Human Services Council; 2020. Accessed May 3, 2024. https://www.chcanys.org/sites/default/files/2020-12/NYS%20SDOH%20Workgroup%20Coding%20Guidance%202020.pdf

36. Massachusetts Medical Society. Case Studies in Social Medicine. *New England Journal of Medicine*. Accessed May 3, 2024. https://www.nejm.org/case-studies-in-social-medicine
37. Social medicine case collection. University of Pittsburgh School of Medicine. Accessed May 3, 2024. https://www.socialmedcases.pitt.edu/?page_id=474
38. Abraham R, Bradley C, Hassan I, Mateja C. Health Disparities Collaborative Subgroup 3: Patient Experience. Alliance for Academic Internal Medicine. Accessed May 3, 2024. https://www.im.org/resources/ume-gme-program-resources/resources-disparities
39. Krishnan A, Rabinowitz M, Ziminsky A, Scott SM, Chretien KC. Addressing race, culture, and structural inequality in medical education: a guide for revising teaching cases. *Acad Med*. 2019;94(4):550–555 PMID: 30640269 doi: 10.1097/acm.0000000000002589
40. Pal D, Taywade M, Gopi K. Experiential learning: how pedagogy is changing in medical education. *Curr Med Issues*. 2022;20(3):198–200 doi: 10.4103/cmi.cmi_35_22
41. Maguire MS, Kottenhahn R, Consiglio-Ward L, Smalls A, Dressler R. Using a poverty simulation in graduate medical education as a mechanism to introduce social determinants of health and cultural competency. *J Grad Med Educ*. 2017;9(3):386–387 PMID: 28638532 doi: 10.4300/JGME-D-16-00776.1
42. Reid CA, Evanson TA. Using simulation to teach about poverty in nursing education: a review of available tools. *J Prof Nurs*. 2016;32(2):130–140 PMID: 27000198 doi: 10.1016/j.profnurs.2015.10.002
43. Jacob SA, Choo Chung CM. Perception of a privilege walk activity and its impact on pharmacy students' views on social justice in a service learning elective: a pilot study. *J Pharm Pract Res*. 2017;47(6):449–456 doi: 10.1002/jppr.1322
44. Wilhite JA, Hardowar K, Fisher H, et al. Clinical problem solving and social determinants of health: a descriptive study using unannounced standardized patients to directly observe how resident physicians respond to social determinants of health. *Diagnosis (Berl)*. 2020;7(3):313–324 PMID: 32735551 doi: 10.1515/dx-2020-0002
45. Hassan I, Kennedy AJ, Agonafer E, et al. Social determinants of health focused home and neighborhood visits: a mixed methods analysis of an internal medicine curriculum. *J Gen Intern Med*. 2023;38(7):1776–1779 PMID: 36451014 doi: 10.1007/s11606-022-07962-y
46. Khan Z, DasGupta S, Krishnamurthy S, Cooper A; Clinical Problem Solvers. *Antiracism in Medicine*. Leveraging narrative medicine to cultivate anti-racist praxis. March 4, 2024. Accessed May 3, 2024. https://clinicalproblemsolving.com/tag/antiracism-in-medicine
47. Kaiser Permanente. *Social Interventions Research & Evaluation Network*. Accessed May 3, 2024. https://sirenetwork.ucsf.edu/siren-podcast
48. Podcasts. *Health Affairs*. Accessed May 3, 2024. https://www.healthaffairs.org/podcasts
49. Metaxas A, Hantgan S, Zwerling J, Desai J, Jariwala SP. The impact of a social media–based educational intervention to promote training in social determinants of health among medical residents. *NeurologyLive*. 2023;6(4)
50. Thistlethwaite JE, Davies D, Ekeocha S, et al. The effectiveness of case-based learning in health professional education. A BEME systematic review: BEME Guide No. 23. *Med Teach*. 2012;34(6):e421–e444 PMID: 22578051 doi: 10.3109/0142159X.2012.680939
51. Fiori KP, Rehm CD, Sanderson D, et al. Integrating social needs screening and community health workers in primary care: the Community Linkage to Care program. *Clin Pediatr (Phila)*. 2020;59(6):547–556 PMID: 32131620 doi: 10.1177/0009922820908589
52. Fiori K, Patel M, Sanderson D, et al. From policy statement to practice: integrating social needs screening and referral assistance with community health workers in an urban academic health center. *J Prim Care Community Health*. 2019;10:2150132719899207 PMID: 31894711 doi: 10.1177/2150132719899207
53. Garg A, Toy S, Tripodis Y, Silverstein M, Freeman E. Addressing social determinants of health at well child care visits: a cluster RCT. *Pediatrics*. 2015;135(2):e296–e304 PMID: 25560448 doi: 10.1542/peds.2014-2888

54. Power-Hays A, Li S, Mensah A, Sobota A. Universal screening for social determinants of health in pediatric sickle cell disease: a quality-improvement initiative. *Pediatr Blood Cancer.* 2020;67(1):e28006 PMID: 31571379 doi: 10.1002/pbc.28006

55. Office of Disease Prevention and Health Promotion. Civic participation. Healthy People 2030. Accessed May 3, 2024. https://health.gov/healthypeople/priority-areas/social-determinants-health/literature-summaries/civic-participation

56. Healthy communities powered by a healthy democracy. Vot-ER. Accessed May 3, 2024. https://vot-er.org

57. Hoffman BD, Rose J, Best D, et al. The Community Pediatrics Training Initiative project planning tool: a practical approach to community-based advocacy. *MedEdPORTAL.* 2017;13:10630 PMID: 30800831 doi: 10.15766/mep_2374-8265.10630

58. Campbell M, Liveris M, Caruso Brown AE, et al. Assessment and evaluation in social determinants of health education: a national survey of US medical schools and physician assistant programs. *J Gen Intern Med.* 2022;37(9):2180–2186 PMID: 35710668 doi: 10.1007/s11606-022-07498-1

59. Hsia SL, Landsfeld A, Lam K, Tuan RL. Implementation and evaluation of a 10-week health equity curriculum for pharmacy students. *Am J Pharm Educ.* 2021;85(9):8579 PMID: 34301552 doi: 10.5688/ajpe8579

60. Orsini MM, Ewald DR, Strack RW. Development and validation of the 4-Factor Critical Consciousness Scale. *SSM Popul Health.* 2022;19:101202 PMID: 36052157 doi: 10.1016/j.ssmph.2022.101202

61. Ross PT, Wiley Cené C, Bussey-Jones J, et al. A strategy for improving health disparities education in medicine. *J Gen Intern Med.* 2010;25(suppl 2):S160–S163 PMID: 20352512 doi: 10.1007/s11606-010-1283-3

CHAPTER 10

Social Determinants of Health in Times of Disruption

Alejandro Hermida, MD, MSc, and Isuree N. Katugampala, MD, MPH

Understanding the social determinants of health (SDOH) compels us to also recognize that these circumstances by which people live and grow are shaped by dynamic forces. These disruptions, such as chronic illness, climate change, migration patterns, pandemics, and economic crises, expose long-standing structural drivers of health inequity. Understanding these disruptions, which people they affect, and what inequity they expose helps health care professionals care for populations vulnerable to these types of disruptions already affected by SDOH in critical ways. This chapter describes the ways in which different disruptions are experienced by populations and how emergencies can dramatically shape people's social, economic, and political futures. By using an adapted ecological systems theory framework to guide this discussion, we seek to explore ways by which individual-, neighborhood-, and population-level disruptions can influence SDOH of populations. We suggest that understanding and addressing SDOH with dynamism is essential in mitigating crises to populations that are caused by emergencies, both locally and globally.

CHAPTER 10

Social Determinants of Health in Times of Disruption

Alejandro Hermida, MD, MSc, and Isuree N. Katugampala, MD, MPH

Introduction

The state of an individual's social well-being is not fixed and can be disrupted in both positive and negative ways. This chapter discusses the effects of scaled disruptions on the way populations experience health and well-being, through the lens of social determinants of health (SDOH). We define *disruption* as an event that changes the socioeconomic landscape in such a way that influences one or more of the SDOH that affect children within the United States. This chapter focuses on specific negative disruptions, such as pandemics, harmful public policies, loss and illness, and climate change, and how they impact SDOH.

Nothing showed more evidence of the importance of addressing SDOH than the COVID-19 pandemic. It exposed the long-standing structural drivers of inequity that affect population health, including both physically and materially precarious working conditions; insufficient wages to afford housing, food, and proper sanitation; and poor access to medical care. This chapter describes the ways in which increasing economic crises, a changing climate, and pandemic-scale disasters can change the socio-politico-economic circumstances of a population. It explains why SDOH cannot be viewed or addressed as a static concept; instead, it relies on dynamism to mitigate unequal exposure to social, economic, environmental, and health risks.

To organize these disruptions, we use an adapted ecological systems theory framework to explore the ways by which individual-, neighborhood-, and population-level disruptions can influence SDOH of populations (**Figure 10-1**). The ecological systems theory organizes the environmental factors that affect a child's development into discrete groups.[1] We use a similar framework to organize the environmental factors that influence the social burden social needs into similar groups. The chapter begins with individual-level disruptions; we discuss the relationship between the SDOH and physical health of a child. We then move forward by discussing microsystem-level disruptions to examine the relationship of a child's immediate surroundings and their s holistic well-being. In using holistic well-being, we are reaffirming the World Health Organization definition of health as a state of "physical, mental and social well-being and not merely the absence of disease or infirmity."[2] The macrosystem-level disruptions are those that occur on a broader societal level. We end by discussing the chronosystem, which looks at the evolving nature of these conditions over time.

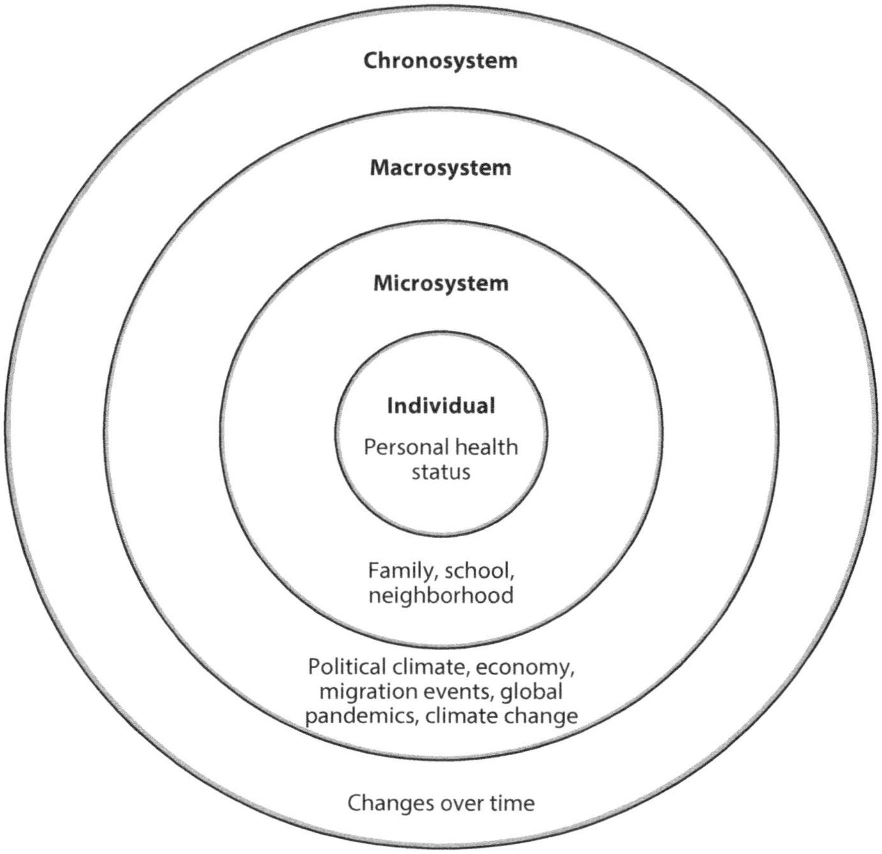

Figure 10-1. Ecological Systems Theory Framework[a]

[a] Of note, the ecological systems theory is more nuanced, with some systems that describe interactions of other systems (eg, the mesosystem and exosystem are where components of the microsystem and macrosystem interact with each other). For the purposes of this chapter, we have simplified our view of this model.

Derived from Bronfenbrenner U. Ecological models of human development. In: *International Encyclopedia of Education.* Vol 3. 2nd ed. Oxford; 1994.

With changing individual and family chronic illness burden, communicable disease emergence, and environmental shifts, child health care professionals face an extraordinary challenge in identifying SDOH needs not only during patient encounters but also between visits and for years, over time. This requires our understanding of the SDOH framework, screening, and response to be dynamic and reflective of our changing world. Understanding how disruptions can manifest in the various planes of a child's life can help build more resilient health care professional responses to SDOH needs.

Individual-Level Disruptions

Personal Health

There is an emerging body of literature that indicates a bidirectional relationship between a child's health and their social well-being. In short, children who experience social burdens tend to have more illness burden, and children with more illness burden are at risk for social burdens. In a cross-sectional study of 56,000 children, Hardy and colleagues found that families that experience higher social needs have less access to primary care and experience higher rates of immediate care services, such as urgent and emergency care encounters.[3] In another study with a similar sample size, families with higher social needs have been shown to be significantly more likely to miss their primary care appointments than families with fewer social needs.[4] Individuals with higher unmet social needs are more likely to exhibit symptoms of depression and engage in risky health behaviors such as using substances.[5] As pediatric providers, we have experienced countless no-shows in primary care settings. In immediate care settings, we have experienced countless encounters in which a child's health has been negatively affected by a preventable illness, or immediate care resources have been required in place of primary care resources that could have been provided in a more cost-effective setting (ie, a pediatrician's office). These families have decreased access, however, and require these safety nets to mitigate the health risks they experience.

A direct link has also been suggested between social burden and increased risk or worsening of chronic health status.[6] Children with chronic medical conditions and unmet social needs are also more likely to use immediate care services than those who have lower social burdens.[7] Children with chronic disabilities are regarded as more vulnerable to changes in family income and housing status and at higher risk for morbidity and mortality related to those shifts. Up to 6 out of every 10 caregivers of children with chronic disabilities have been shown to report an unmet social need.[8] Certain chronic conditions, such as obesity and asthma, are more often reported in children who live in public housing.[9] Although these studies show correlation and not necessarily causation, a direct relationship can be inferred—a relationship in which a decline in physical health begets a decline in socioeconomic well-being and in which a decline in socioeconomic well-being begets a decline in physical health.

Key Concept

Families with higher individual health needs, such as chronic illness burden, may experience higher social need burdens.

Microsystem-Level Disruptions

There is growing evidence regarding disruptions to individuals' family structures and neighborhood safety that contribute to their social and economic well-being. Next, we discuss the impacts of caregiver death, family separation in the context of immigration status and child welfare, and gun violence as examples of this disruption to SDOH across age ranges.

Caregiver Loss

The loss of a parent or caregiver is linked to a higher risk for mental health issues and is comorbid with symptoms of anxiety and depression. This event can lead to a feeling of loss of control, suicidality, concentration or behavioral issues in school, and inability to meet goals toward one's future. This disruption in the family unit can lead to children or adolescents being raised by another family member, which may cause additional stressors, including increased financial burden for the new caregiver, reduced time and support to the child who has experienced loss, and difficulty adjusting to the new circumstance.[10] This ripple effect, not only through an individual's mental well-being but also through the individual's network of family, relatives, and peers, shows how this type of disruption affects the social fabric and economic well-being of many others embedded within this life event.

Regarding how to address this level of disruption, studies have shown that even brief supportive interventions can help prevent children and adolescents from experiencing severe mental health issues after caregiver loss.[10] Findings from these studies show that support groups for new caregivers and children affected by loss can improve outcomes in mental health in children and caregivers.

Family Separation

Political policies related to the separation of children from their caregivers, including separation in times of crisis, have palpable impacts on the family unit. Through changing political climates, some immigration policies have led to families experiencing separation, deportation, and economic hardship. Research done among Latino/Latina adolescents regarding deportation of a family member shows that the consequences of these policies have led to increased suicidal ideation, alcohol use at a young age, and a host of externalizing symptoms.[11] The separation of a family member through deportation, for example, can lead to income loss, housing instability, food insecurity, schooling interruptions, marginalization, and social isolation.[11] This finding underscores that anti-immigrant policies have deleterious impacts on children and related family members.

Child welfare proceedings and outcomes can also disrupt family structure. Racially disproportionate rates of child welfare cases, from abuse and neglect investigations to parental terminations, also contribute to mental health and socioeconomic outcomes of Black families and their children. For example, in California, nearly half of all Black children and their families have experienced investigation by child protective services.[12] When children are removed from the home, many parents or caregivers receive reduced benefits for food assistance or housing or have their wages garnished to pay foster care providers, exacerbating poverty and therefore making it more difficult for parents/caregivers to make the case to reunify with their children.[12] Children and adults who have experienced the child welfare system and foster care system report poor outcomes in mental health, educational interruptions, and chronic mental health and substance use issues as a result of their separation and out-of-home placements.[12]

Separation and detention of children from their caregivers is another example of political policy leading to parental attachment issues, economic hardship, and poor educational outcomes. Studies of separated children in immigrant households show increased suicidality, anxiety, and psychological distress.[13] This heightened amount of psychological stress can increase the burden of chronic disease among individuals who have experienced separation and may worsen educational outcomes.[13]

To mitigate some of these negative outcomes, strengthening the community system has shown to play an essential role in improving relationships between family members and increasing their sense of belonging. We suggest promoting engagement in school and helping families enroll in school, as all newly arrived children are entitled to free public education in the United States. In addition, health care professionals can help families navigate complex immigration and child welfare policies.

Gun Violence

The incidence of gun violence has increased, leading to disruptions in community structures and an overall sense of safety. Those who have experienced school shootings are at risk for posttraumatic stress surrounding the school environment, disrupting the sense of community.[14] Higher poverty levels correlate with higher deaths from firearms throughout the United States.[14] The disproportionate lack of mental health resources in impoverished communities are immediately exacerbated in these communities. In addition, the increased firearm mortality rates may contribute to disproportionate burden of violence on some racial and ethnic groups.[14] The interconnectedness of this issue of violence with economic hardship illustrates how by integrating SDOH into our health encounters, health care professionals can participate in mitigating gun violence.

Key Concept

Changes in the family unit, through caregiver death or family separation, are strongly related to a variety of SDOH: poverty and mental health exacerbations. Gun violence and family separation are experienced disproportionately in populations with higher social needs.

Macrosystem-Level Disruptions

Next, we suggest that the macrosystem be used to represent the sociopolitical contexts that influence the microsystem of a child—specifically, how policies, the economy, climate change, and global pandemics have affected the social well-being of children and the family units they belong to.

Political and Economic Crises

Because the success of the economy is directly tied to employment, wages, housing, and costs of goods, it has significant impacts on how care is sought and how well-being is attained. Food and housing insecurity also increase dramatically in times of recession. For example, the global economic recession of 2008 led to soaring unemployment rates, inflation, and stagnant wages. These impacts only deepen those of social factors on the physical health of a community. The American Recovery and Reinvestment Act signed in 2009 sought to address this, by funding programs to support those affected by job loss, through the Supplemental Nutrition Assistance Program, housing supports, and unemployment benefits.[15] Although a recession affects those across the class and wealth spectrum, these effects are magnified for people with low incomes or from racial and ethnic groups that have been marginalized. Black and Hispanic individuals are overrepresented in the industries that experience the highest unemployment rates.[15] These communities are also less able to afford food, housing, and health care than their white counterparts. In this way, physical health is indirectly affected by the decline of their social well-being during economic crises. This indirect relation to health is not singular; economic recessions also have direct impacts on health.

The United States has one of the few political systems that ties health care to employment. In economic recessions, when unemployment rates rise, there are significant losses of health care coverage for many US residents. This was central in the 2008 Great Recession, where it became a centerpiece of political discussion in the presidential and local government debates. Former President Barack Obama's administration drafted the Affordable Care Act, which sought to mitigate the lack of access to health care that disproportionately affected lower socioeconomic status and minority groups throughout the country. Although its structure was elaborate and improved the rate of uninsurance among low-income populations, the complexities in policy rendered it vulnerable to attacks, thereby limiting its full impact. It remains clear that investment in health care, insurance, and the funding of public policy measures helps improve health outcomes across race, class, and gender.

International Migration and Conflicts

Although the goal of this chapter is to distill the impacts of disrupted SDOH on individuals within the United States, it is imperative to understand the patterns of migration, including the reasons for immigration and seeking refuge across the world and international political crisis. Migration journeys have increased worldwide, and individuals are often compelled to leave their home countries for survival, safety, and employment. While what is experienced within migrants' respective countries can drastically differ from what is experienced within the United States, the events migrants encounter as a part of their migration and within their integration into the United States drastically affect health and social and economic well-being.[16,17] Oftentimes, immigration is both a consequence of SDOH in a home country and can be considered an SDOH, as it changes the needs of people once they arrive in the United States.

People who are immigrants have specific and unique SDOH profiles. In many cases, immigrant groups have some of the greatest social burden in a given community, given the acuity of their needs and lack of social support.[16] In times of international conflict, political crisis, or economic crisis, immigrant populations may increase dramatically, especially in so-called sanctuary cities.[17] This increase can lead directly to strains on public and community resource groups. As health care professionals, it is crucial to understand the different needs faced by immigrant populations, not only in the health consequences of their journey but also in the landscape by which these high-needs populations find and build their lives in a new home. By working with community groups that advocate for increased local resources when immigration rates are higher, we believe that health care professionals can better participate in the holistic well-being of immigrant populations.

Climate and Environmental Disruptions

Climate change poses an important threat to our collective well-being. While the topic has been debated on political stages to a significantly higher extent than in academic settings, we are now beginning to see tangible effects on human health caused by climate changes. Human behavior is directly influenced by rising temperatures. One study from the National Bureau of Economic Research revealed higher rates of homicide in warmer months compared to cooler months.[18] These changes were more pronounced in lower-income neighborhoods, which only aggravates the economic divide between social classes.

Climate change has more pervasive negative effects beyond human behavior. Changes in temperature, precipitation patterns, and extreme weather events influence the agricultural food chain supply, which in turn increases food insecurity.[19] Sea levels are predicted to rise, affecting the international seaports through which the United States obtains a significant portion of its food supply.[19] Those in higher-income communities likely have more chance of adapting to these changes.[20] Those in lower-income communities, however, are more likely to reside in floodplains or live in housing that is less resilient to extreme weather conditions.[20] Families living in high-risk zones are less likely to have appropriate insurance, and families of color are even less likely to have insurance. These communities also experience higher rates of displacement. Although national support exists to respond to these events, there are systemic racial and social inequities in federal assistance, such as Federal Emergency Management Agency interventions, offered during these weather events.[20] Research indicates that white families are likely to get higher reimbursement than Black and Hispanic families for property damages. One study showed that the mean reimbursement rate for white families was $126,000 compared to approximately $28,000 for Black and Hispanic families following an extreme weather event.[20]

Extreme weather events are displacing families. In the southwestern United States, where fires have increased in frequency and intensity, families have not only been displaced but also been left with insufficient resources to adapt and treat the mental and emotional effects of their losses. For those who are not directly affected by these events, repeated media exposures to extreme weather events have been shown to increase stress levels and to increase mental health risks, indicating that climate change may have a direct impact on the disparities in mental health.[19]

Climate changes have the potential to lead to increases in secondary toxic runoff from factories, increases in fires leading to particulate matter generation and poor air quality, and increases in displacement caused by rising sea levels.[21] The resulting impacts on the health of children and their families can include a rise in blood lead levels, an increase in asthma-related morbidity and mortality, and the loss of a home from flooding and rising flood insurance costs, requiring families to move from their homes.[19,20] Climate changes expose the tangible connection between health and the physical environment. As pediatricians, we should understand how to respond to climate disasters and their secondary effects on the social and physical well-being of children and families.

Global Pandemics

Pandemics throughout history have exposed vulnerabilities in our socioeconomic fabric. The COVID-19 pandemic was no different in that regard, with widespread loss of life and livelihood for so many. It required swift response in community-level changes, policy-level changes, and biomedical-level changes. Although the next pandemic cannot be predicted, we can expect similar global diseases to occur again, which will require responses that consider health not only as the biological well-being of an individual and populations but also as the complete social, economic, and mental well-being of the individual and populations.

By 2023, the Centers for Disease Control and Prevention data have shown that in the United States alone, more than 1 million people have died of COVID-19 and its complications.[22] While this death toll is significant in sheer number, additionally, it speaks to the impact in terms of the people and communities left behind. Social determinants of health screening efforts during the pandemic showed that there was a significant increase in needs identified; however, there is often limited access to resources and longer waiting times post-pandemic.[23] In New York City, food insecurity rates rose for children and their families, as schools that provided free or reduced-cost meals could no longer do so because of the shift to online learning.[24] Studies conducted in the Bronx, NY, which was heavily affected by COVID-19 in 2020 to 2021, demonstrated a significant increase in housing quality issues, food insecurity, and legal needs.[23] Physical distancing measures were integral in stopping the spread of COVID-19 but were substantially difficult in communities with high rates of populations that were unhoused.[24] Internet access was also crucial for coordinating unemployment insurance, schooling, and telehealth appointments, but it was a major challenge for those in rural areas who faced issues with reliable high-speed internet access.[24] The COVID-19 pandemic demonstrated higher mortality among those with higher SDOH needs, particularly in low-income areas and those with a high proportion of Black population.[25] In the United States, the COVID-19 pandemic exacerbated inequalities not only in the form of mortality but also in the form of disruptions to resources, social networks, and housing.[26]

The COVID-19 pandemic also highlighted low wages and poor working conditions as other structural drivers of inequity. Major illness outbreaks were recorded in slaughterhouses and other places of employment that were deemed essential during the pandemic but provided low income.[26] Because of the economic instability within families, many workers risked going to work with illness, leading to massive outbreaks.[26] Immigration status may have also played a role, as some workers may have felt pressured to work in unsafe environments, without proper workplace distancing protections, because they feared losing employment.[26] These findings show the connection between structural and institutional racism, class division, and immigration status and health, causing deleterious results for individuals and populations. In the United States, child tax credit (CTC) payments lessened the disruptions felt by many during the COVID-19 pandemic.[27]

Key Concept

Large-scale disruptions in the sociopolitical and physical landscape (eg, pandemics, climate change, immigration crises) have been shown to exacerbate the social needs in a variety of populations. These disruptions warrant adaptive changes in how we address social needs.

Chronosystem and Addressing Social Determinants in Times of Disruptions

The chronosystem is the final layer of the ecological systems theory, which suggests that time also influences health and well-being. The social burden for a given population, for better or for worse, can change over time. All the themes discussed in this chapter exist within this concept. Weather events, global pandemics, and international crises may increase or decrease in frequency over time. But positive changes can also occur. During the COVID-19 pandemic, there was a surge of autonomous community groups that mobilized to address food and housing insecurity, and enhancements to the Special Supplemental Nutrition Program for Women, Infants, and Children; Early Intervention Program; and CTC decreased the gap in health disparities among children, which helped build needed safety nets to address SDOH within a wider context.[27]

Key Concept

Disruptions are not fixed in time and are subject to change. Understanding historical examples of disruptions should inform how we address current and future fluctuations in the disruptions that persist and newly arise.

Key Points

- Social determinants of health are not a static concept; they fluctuate in response to changes in personal, political, social, economic, and physical environments.
- Understanding past fluctuations in people's social, political, economic, and personal well-being helps us understand how the SDOH framework can be applied to future disruptions.
- Disruptions in the family or school environment negatively affect the social landscape of children.
- As climate change hastens and its effects on global pandemics, migration patterns, and food shortages become evident, populations experience exacerbations of social, economic, and health needs.
- Because of the evolving nature of SDOH, solutions to issues in times of disruption require the ability to change.

References

1. Brofenbrenner U. *Ecological Models of Human Development*. Vol 3. 2nd ed. International Encyclopedia of Education; 1993
2. Schramme T. Health as complete well-being: the WHO definition and beyond. *Public Health Ethics*. 2023;16(3):210–218 PMID: 38333767 doi: 10.1093/phe/phad017
3. Hardy R, Boch S, Keedy H, Chisolm D. Social determinants of health needs and pediatric health care use. *J Pediatr*. 2021;238:275–281.e1 PMID: 34329688 doi: 10.1016/j.jpeds.2021.07.056
4. Fiori KP, Heller CG, Rehm CD, et al. Unmet social needs and no-show visits in primary care in a US northeastern urban health system, 2018–2019. *Am J Public Health*. 2020;110(suppl 2):S242–S250 PMID: 32663075 doi: 10.2105/AJPH.2020.305717
5. Cockerham WC, Hamby BW, Oates GR. Social determinants of chronic disease. *Am J Prev Med*. 2017;52(1)(suppl 1):S5–S12 PMID: 27989293 doi: 10.1016/j.amepre.2016.09.010
6. Heller CG, Rehm CD, Parsons AH, Chambers EC, Hollingsworth NH, Fiori KP. The association between social needs and chronic conditions in a large, urban primary care population. *Prev Med*. 2021;153:106752 PMID: 34348133 doi: 10.1016/j.ypmed.2021.106752
7. Foster CC, Simon TD, Qu P, et al. Social determinants of health and emergency and hospital use by children with chronic disease. *Hosp Pediatr*. 2020;10(6):471–480 PMID: 32423995 doi: 10.1542/hpeds.2019-0248
8. Brehaut JC, Kohen DE, Garner RE, et al. Health among caregivers of children with health problems: findings from a Canadian population-based study. *Am J Public Health*. 2009;99(7):1254–1262 PMID: 19059861 doi: 10.2105/AJPH.2007.129817
9. Chambers EC, Heller C, Fiori K, McAuliff K, Rehm CD. Chronic pediatric health conditions among youth living in public housing and receiving care in a large hospital system in Bronx, NY. *Glob Pediatr Health*. 2020;7:2333794X20971164 PMID: 33241085 doi: 10.1177/2333794X20971164
10. Bergman AS, Axberg U, Hanson E. When a parent dies—a systematic review of the effects of support programs for parentally bereaved children and their caregivers. *BMC Palliat Care*. 2017;16(1):39 PMID: 28797262 doi: 10.1186/s12904-017-0223-y
11. Roche KM, White RMB, Lambert SF, et al. Association of family member detention or deportation with Latino or Latina adolescents' later risks of suicidal ideation, alcohol use, and externalizing problems. *JAMA Pediatr*. 2020;174(5):478–486 PMID: 32176245 doi: 10.1001/jamapediatrics.2020.0014

12. Naveed H, Neier A. "If I wasn't poor, I wouldn't be unfit": the family separation crisis in the US child welfare system. Human Rights Watch. November 17, 2022. Accessed May 6, 2024. https://www.hrw.org/report/2022/11/17/if-i-wasnt-poor-i-wouldnt-be-unfit/family-separation-crisis-us-child-welfare#1300
13. Linton JM, Griffin M, Shapiro AJ; American Academy of Pediatrics Council on Community Pediatrics. Detention of immigrant children. *Pediatrics*. 2017;139(5):e20170483 PMID: 28289140 doi: 10.1542/peds.2017-0483
14. Roberts BK, Nofi CP, Cornell E, Kapoor S, Harrison L, Sathya C. Trends and disparities in firearm deaths among children. *Pediatrics*. 2023;152(3):e2023061296 PMID: 37599647 doi: 10.1542/peds.2023-061296
15. Backhaus I, Hoven H, Di Tecco C, Iavicoli S, Conte A, Dragano N. Economic change and population health: lessons learnt from an umbrella review on the Great Recession. *BMJ Open*. 2022;12(4):e060710 PMID: 35379647 doi: 10.1136/bmjopen-2021-060710
16. Castañeda H, Holmes SM, Madrigal DS, Young ME, Beyeler N, Quesada J. Immigration as a social determinant of health. *Annu Rev Public Health*. 2015;36:375–392 PMID: 25494053 doi: 10.1146/annurev-publhealth-032013-182419
17. Perreira KM, Pedroza JM. Policies of exclusion: implications for the health of immigrants and their children. *Annu Rev Public Health*. 2019;40:147–166 PMID: 30601722 doi: 10.1146/annurev-publhealth-040218-044115
18. Asher J. A rise in murder? let's talk about the weather. *New York Times*. September 21, 2018. Accessed May 6, 2024. https://www.nytimes.com/2018/09/21/upshot/a-rise-in-murder-lets-talk-about-the-weather.html
19. Ragavan MI, Marcil LE, Garg A. Climate change as a social determinant of health. *Pediatrics*. 2020;145(5):e20193169 PMID: 32265296 doi: 10.1542/peds.2019-3169
20. Howell J, Elliott JR. Damages done: the longitudinal impacts of natural hazards on wealth inequality in the United States. *Soc Probl*. 2019;66(3):448–467 doi: 10.1093/socpro/spy016
21. Ahdoot S, Baum CR, Cataletto MB, Hogan P, Wu CB, Bernstein A; American Academy of Pediatrics Council on Environmental Health and Climate Change; Council on Children and Disasters; Section on Pediatric Pulmonology and Sleep Medicine; and Section on Minority Health, Equity, and Inclusion. Climate change and children's health: building a healthy future for every child. *Pediatrics*. 2024;153(3):e2023065504 PMID: 38374809 doi: 10.1542/peds.2023-065504
22. Centers for Disease Control and Prevention. COVID Data Tracker. Accessed October 21, 2024. https://covid.cdc.gov/covid-data-tracker/#datatracker-home
23. Azan A, Stephens J, Xie X, Fiori K, Gover M. COVID-19 and changes in reported social risk factors at a primary care practice in the South Bronx. *J Prim Care Community Health*. 2023;14:21501319221147136 PMID: 36625253 doi: 10.1177/21501319221147136
24. Brakefield WS, Olusanya OA, White B, Shaban-Nejad A. Social determinants and indicators of COVID-19 among marginalized communities: a scientific review and call to action for pandemic response and recovery. *Disaster Med Public Health Prep*. 2022;17:e193 PMID: 35492024 doi: 10.1017/dmp.2022.104
25. Dalsania AK, Fastiggi MJ, Kahlam A, et al. The relationship between social determinants of health and racial disparities in COVID-19 mortality. *J Racial Ethn Health Disparities*. 2022;9(1):288–295 PMID: 33403652 doi: 10.1007/s40615-020-00952-y
26. Paremoer L, Nandi S, Serag H, Baum F. COVID-19 pandemic and the social determinants of health. *BMJ*. 2021;372(129):n129 PMID: 33509801 doi: 10.1136/bmj.n129
27. McCann NC, Dean LT, Bovell-Ammon A, et al. Association between Child Tax Credit advance payments and food insufficiency in households experiencing economic shocks. *Health Aff Sch*. 2024;2(2):qxae011 PMID: 38756550 doi: 10.1093/haschl/qxae011

CHAPTER 11

Policy Reform, Movement Toward Universal Social Needs Screening, and Future Directions

Jana C. Leary, MD, MS, and Arvin Garg, MD, MPH, FAAP

Pediatric clinicians can make a positive impact on some of the adverse social determinants of health that patients face. At the practice level amid recent policy reforms, we can implement family-centered social needs screening and referral strategies that are tailored to the pediatric setting. We do not need to start from scratch in these efforts; rather, we can leverage available screening tools, referral platforms, and implementation toolkits, as well as forge partnerships with community-based organizations to strengthen the social care we provide to our patients and families. Looking to the future, we can also think creatively about how to use information technology innovations in our screening and referral efforts to improve reach, efficiency, and effectiveness. Ultimately, no matter which approach a clinic or an institution takes to social needs screening and referral, we must strive to do so with an anti-racist lens. We must take the time to explain the universal nature of screening and our intent to understand patients' lived experiences so we can provide equitable care. If we demonstrate empathy, humility, and non-judgment throughout this process, we may avoid unintended consequences from screening, strengthen our therapeutic relationships with caregivers and patients, and destigmatize social services.

CHAPTER 11

Policy Reform, Movement Toward Universal Social Needs Screening, and Future Directions

Jana C. Leary, MD, MS, and Arvin Garg, MD, MPH, FAAP

Introduction

With the high burden of poverty in the United States, many children are affected by adverse social determinants of health (SDOH) and unmet social needs that can have negative effects on children's physical and mental health throughout the entirety of their life courses. We must make federal, state, practice, and individual-level efforts to prevent or alleviate the effects of adverse SDOH and promote child health and health equity. In this chapter, we will discuss such efforts through policy, policy reform, and the movement toward universal social needs screening and referral within health care as well as potential future directions for social care within clinical settings.

The Social Safety Net, Politics, and Policy Reform

Globally, children are more likely to live in poverty than adults. According to UNICEF, it is estimated that more than 350 million children live in extreme poverty worldwide.[1] Despite being the wealthiest country in the world by net worth, the United States has greater child poverty than most countries with similar resource profiles and wealth. According to US Census data using the Supplemental Poverty Measure, the US child poverty rate is rising at a rapid pace, more than doubling from 5.2% in 2021 to 12.4% in 2022 (**Figure 11-1**).[2]

Although this reality may seem bleak, another reality is positive and certain—that state and federal investments in supporting families with supplemental income and/or public benefits for basic needs such as food, along with investments in the broader social safety net, can reduce child poverty rates and in turn improve child health. Safety net resources, and their effects on child poverty and health, shrink and grow depending on our current political landscape.

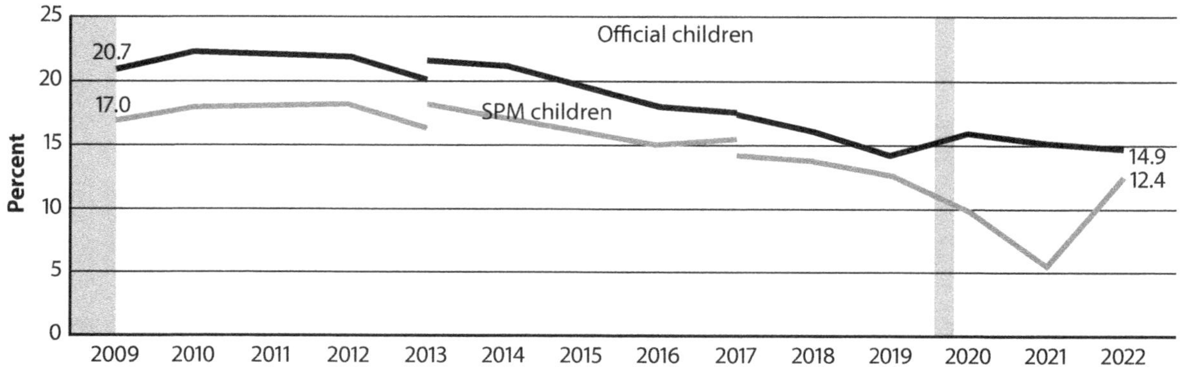

Figure 11-1. Child Poverty Rates Using the Official and Supplemental Poverty Measure: 2009 to 2022

Official includes unrelated individuals under the age of 15. SPM indicates Supplemental Poverty Measure.

From Shrider EA, Creamer J. Poverty in the United States: 2022. US Census Bureau. September 12, 2023. Accessed May 6, 2024. https://www.census.gov/library/publications/2023/demo/p60-280.html.

Exemplar Safety Net Programs

According to the American Academy of Pediatrics (AAP) policy statement "Poverty and Child Heath in the United States," longitudinal studies performed from the 1960s to 2012 demonstrated that government programs providing income supports and direct social benefits cut the poverty rate for families with children nearly in half, from a projected rate of 31% to an actual rate of 18%.[3]

Tax policies such as the Earned Income Tax Credit (EITC) and the Child Tax Credit (CTC), implemented at federal and state levels, have effectively incentivized employment and supplemented income for families working at low wages. Research has estimated that the federal EITC alone lifted more than 3 million children out of poverty by the early 2000s and improved infant health with higher rates of prenatal care and lower rates of preterm birth and low birth weight.[4] During the COVID-19 pandemic, the CTC was expanded to extend full refundability to families with little or no taxable income. The 2021 CTC expansion caused an immediate reduction in child poverty (**Figure 11-2**), reaching a historically low rate of 5.2%[5]; studies demonstrated that the CTC funds were used effectively to meet families' most basic needs. To learn more about EITC and CTC, refer to Chapter 5, Financial Assistance and Access to Care.

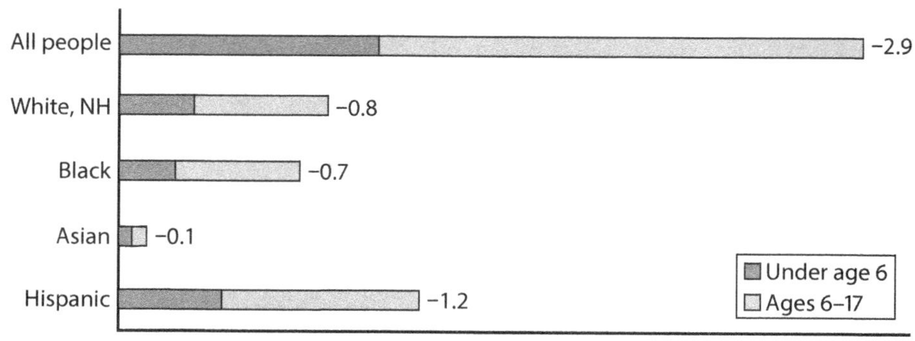

Figure 11-2. Change in the Number of Children in Poverty (in Millions) in Response to the Child Tax Credit: 2021

NH indicates non-Hispanic.

From Burns K, Fox L, Wilson D. Expansions to Child Tax Credit contributed to 46% decline in child poverty since 2020. US Census Bureau. September 13, 2022. Accessed May 6, 2024. https://www.census.gov/library/stories/2022/09/record-drop-in-child-poverty.html.

Programs focused on raising the minimum wage have also been shown to lift children out of poverty and improve child health and development. Such programs provide families with greater income stability, allowing them to obtain needs of daily living, such as food or housing, more consistently. Research has shown that increasing family income, even by just a few thousand dollars annually, can increase child math and reading performance and improve SAT scores.[6]

Key Concept

Government investments that provide supplemental income or public benefits for basic needs such as food and housing for families, or that contribute to the broader social safety net, are effective in decreasing child poverty rates and improving child health. These resources and their effects on child health shift with the political landscape in the United States.

Other federally funded programs focused on increasing child health care access, education, and nutritional supports have also made major impacts on child health. The Children's Health Insurance Program decreased the rate of uninsurance among children in families with low-incomes by 70% and increased access to preventive medical care.[3,7] Early childhood interventions such as Head Start and Early Head Start, providing child care and educational services for low-income families, have been shown to improve child cognitive functioning, self-regulation, and development.[3] The Supplemental Nutrition Program for Women, Infants, and Children (WIC) and Supplemental Nutrition Assistance Program (SNAP), which provide nutritional support for pregnant and postpartum women and people, young children, and low-income families, have been shown to reduce poverty, preterm birth, and infant mortality rates and to improve child mental and cognitive development.[3,8] To learn more about WIC and SNAP, refer to Chapter 7, Food Insecurity.

To continue to make forward strides in addressing child poverty, we will need federal and state investments to develop and maintain more social care policy interventions such as these. Political shifts that reduce funding for social care of children will have deleterious effects on child health and development. Regardless of our political stance, to optimize children's health and development, we as clinicians must advocate for policies that will invest in and support a robust social safety net for families.

Policy Reform

Perhaps the largest policy reform of the modern era that was meant to focus national attention on the importance of the SDOH and the social safety net was the Affordable Care Act (ACA, colloquially referred to as "Obamacare") in 2010. The ACA had 3 primary goals:

- To increase the availability of affordable health insurance for US inhabitants
- To expand Medicaid coverage to more individuals
- To facilitate new health care delivery methods designed to lower health care costs

The ACA supported the creation of accountable care organizations (ACOs).[9] An ACO is a group of physicians, other health care professionals, and hospitals that form a partnership to deliver care to its members, improve population health, and control health care costs. The ACO approach deviated from previous models of care delivery in its emphasis on the importance of individualized care to meet patients' unique needs, better coordination of health care services, and attention to health-related SDOH. For example, ACOs are required to complete a Care Needs Screening, including specific screening for social needs, for new members within 90 days of joining the ACO. These screening requirements facilitate early identification of members with social needs for which the ACO then conducts a comprehensive assessment and creates an individualized care plan to address those needs.

An ACO is incentivized to screen for social needs, not only to meet its goal of providing higher quality and individualized health care to its members as previously described but also to maximize financial returns through Medicaid's risk-adjusted payments. Accountable care organizations that care for members with greater needs, including both medical and social needs, receive higher payments.

Key Concept

Policy reform such as the ACA focused national attention on the importance of SDOH. This heightened attention and associated shift in care and payment models encouraged creation of standardized screening tools and referral interventions that can support clinician efforts in addressing patients' social needs, in turn improving health.

This paradigm shift in care and payment models caused a cascade of downstream effects, including the creation of more standardized social needs screening tools, implementation toolkits, referral platforms, and other referral interventions to address identified social needs. Within pediatric ambulatory care, standardized social needs screening and referral is becoming routine practice and has been shown to effectively identify families in need who may benefit from social resources; increase family connections to community, state, and federal resources; and improve parent-reported child health and immunization rates.[10–15] Although social needs screening and referral may be relatively less commonplace in pediatric inpatient settings, when the process is performed, studies have demonstrated benefits such as increased family connections to social service professionals and community resource information and improved parental opinion of the physicians' role in social care.[16–19]

Reform Affecting Pediatric Inpatient Care

From 2023 onward, we have been seeing a large uptick in performance of pediatric inpatient social needs screening and referral distribution. This is, in part, because in January 2023, multiple standard-setting organizations, including The Joint Commission (TJC), the National Committee for Quality Assurance (NCQA), and the Centers for Medicare & Medicaid Services (CMS), launched national quality initiatives that require incorporation of screening for social needs, some also requiring incorporation of referral interventions, into routine inpatient medical care.[20] In the early phase of these initiatives, hospitals' inpatient social needs screening and referral performance will not have any associated financial accountability. But that is likely to change over time, becoming a standard quality outcome metric, with financial return also becoming an incentive for hospitals to develop and implement inpatient social needs screening and referral programs.

At the initial launch of these national social care quality measures and regulations in 2023, each standard-setting agency (ie, TJC, NCQA, CMS) varied in its recommended approach to inpatient social needs screening and referral (eg, which social domains to screen; which screening tool to use, if any; which populations to screen; and whether an associated referral intervention is required). For some social care experts, this variation raised concern that the new inpatient standards were potentially launched prematurely, without the depth of inpatient-specific research and development of inpatient-specific tools required to ensure that inpatient social care programs would be beneficial and make meaningful improvements to child health and health equity.[20] More time and research will be required to determine the ultimate impact that inpatient social needs screening may have on child health outcomes.

Implementing Social Care Systems Across a Variety of Clinical Settings

Given the burden of poverty in the United states, the resultant policy reforms, requirements from standard-setting organizations, and policy statements by the AAP and the American Academy of Family Physicians (AAFP) recommending screening for and addressing unmet social needs at all child health visits, we are likely to see a massive increase in the implementation of social care programs within various clinical care settings, expanding at a rapid pace with the goal to be universal practice.[20–22]

Implementation Science: Consideration of Contextual Facilitators and Barriers

Implementing social needs screening and referral systems more broadly, across many different clinical environments, will not be an easy task. Every clinical site's patient population and workflow are unique, with contextual facilitators and barriers that must be considered for implementation to be most successful. An implementation strategy that works for screening and referral at one ambulatory clinic, for example, may not work within the workflows and resource constraints of a clinic right down the hallway within the same building. What works within several ambulatory clinics may not work at all or may require significant adaptation to work within an inpatient setting. Considering these issues through the lens of implementation science, a one-size-fits-all approach simply will not work.[23] When attempting to expand implementation efforts and integrate them into routine practice within a variety of clinical settings, is it essential that each site take the time to engage key groups including families, clinicians, and community partners to consider its own unique context, facilitators, and personnel that can be leveraged for screening and addressing social needs and its own unique barriers that must be overcome for implementation to be successful (**Figure 11-3**). This planning and development stage is not easy, but it is essential. If we fail to take adequate time to consider our facilitators and barriers and to develop unique implementation strategies tailored to our own environments, implementation of social needs screening and referral may not achieve maximal benefits for families. Or worse, in the context of suboptimal implementation, our efforts could even be harmful for families if we create expectations for social support that we are not ultimately able to provide. If implementation strategies are not developed to maximize fit and appropriateness within each unique clinical environment, even the most well-meaning implementation efforts are likely to fizzle out entirely over time.

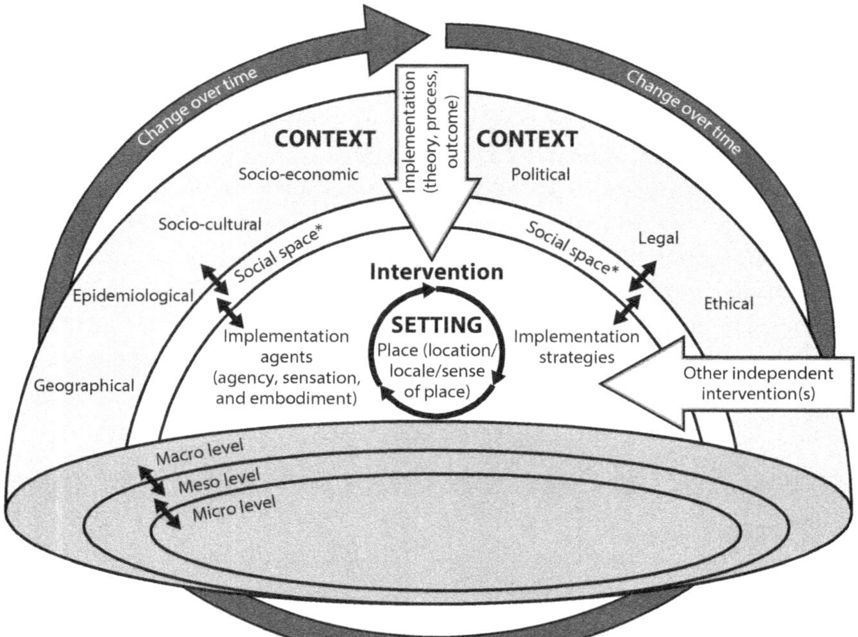

Figure 11-3. Considering Unique Context, Facilitators, and Barriers in Implementing Complex Interventions: The Adapted Context and Implementation of Complex Interventions (CICI) Framework

Adapted CICI framework based on identified concepts (marked with *).

From Mielke J, De Geest S, Zúñiga F, et al. Understanding dynamic complexity in context-enriching contextual analysis in implementation science from a constructivist perspective. *Front Health Serv.* 2022;2:953731.

Key Concept

When trying to implement social needs screening and referral across a variety of clinical settings, with a spectrum of available resources, a one-size-fits-all approach will not work. Engaging essential personnel and considering each clinic's or institution's unique facilitators and barriers to screening for and addressing needs will be paramount to develop implementation strategies that are effective and sustainable over time.

Building From Existing Resources

When considering where to start when building our clinical sites' unique social needs screening and referral implementation strategies, it may feel overwhelming. It's important to note, however, that we need not start from scratch. Many clinical, research, and social care leaders have worked hard to create and test a variety of standardized social needs screening tools, such as the Well Child Care, Evaluation, Community Resources, Advocacy, Referral, Education (WE CARE) screening tool; Health Leads questionnaire; Protocol for Responding to and Assessing Patients' Assets, Risks and Experience (PRAPARE); Accountable Health Communities screening tool; and I-HELP questions, among many others, that we can use or adapt to fit our specific populations and settings.[11,24–27] (For a summary of the screening tools mentioned, refer to Table 4-1 of Chapter 4, Screening for Social Needs in the Pediatric Clinical Setting.) Multiple online and technology-based referral platforms have been built and tested (eg, FindHelp, Unite Us, Neighborhood Navigator) that can assist with referral to social resources.[28,29] Of course, we must again consider if and how each of these platforms would fit into our particular environments (eg, electronic health record [EHR] compatibility, catchment population, platform cost) and that they may not be the best approach for all.

Standard-setting organizations have also created social care toolkits to which clinicians can refer when considering how to build their sites' implementation strategies. For example, The EveryONE Project Toolkit from the AAFP is a one-stop shop for implicit bias and health equity education and training, social needs screening tools, resource referrals by zip code, and tips for community engagement.[29] The Social Interventions Research & Evaluation Network (SIREN) provides an entire Evidence and Research Library, allowing clinicians to see the evidence behind developed tools and to easily access digestible summary documents such as its *Community Resource Referral Platforms* guide and screening tool comparison tables (**Figure 11-4**).[28,30] SIREN resources can facilitate efficient perusal of available social needs screening and referral options, which may help clinicians develop their own site's specific implementation strategies or spark ideas for innovative new options.

Working Within Resource Constraints

Even with the building blocks and tools described to facilitate social needs screening and referral, real-world implementation can be particularly difficult in clinical settings in which resources and personnel required for performing screening and/or responding to social needs are sparse. Clinical practices from the same region could consider banding together, forming an alliance for social care, and sharing resources and workload required for screening and referral.

It is also important to remember that our local community-based organizations (CBOs) are experts on social care and have worked in this area far longer than any health care entity. Clinical practices should consider forming and/or formalizing partnerships with their local community health workers (CHWs) and CBOs to facilitate referrals to relevant resources and potentiate more longitudinal social care for children and their families.

Unintended Consequences

Good intentions are the foundation and the primary motivation for pediatric practitioners to perform social needs screening and referral. Clinicians routinely ask parents and caregivers about adverse social circumstances out of a desire and intention to help, knowing intuitively the impact that the social environment has on children's ability to thrive. But screening for social needs is inherently different from traditional screening for medical problems to which clinicians are more accustomed. If a patient screens positively for a medical problem, clinicians can respond with interventions including treatments and medications that are readily accessible. In contrast, the services and social resources required to potentially alleviate a detected unmet social need are beyond the scope of traditional clinical training and clinical care.

In this context, there is potential for unintended harm, despite the good intentions and potential benefits of screening for and addressing social needs.[31] Clinicians may be uncomfortable asking about sensitive social issues such as food insecurity or interpersonal violence, as traditional medical training does not provide instruction on how to compassionately ask about and respond to social concerns raised, particularly in front of children and/or other family members.

Features	Aunt Bertha	CharityTracker	CrossTx	Healthify	NowPow	One Degree	Pieces Iris	TAVConnect	Unite Us
Version	Enterprise Platform	CharityTracker	CrossTx	Coordinate	PowRx	One Degree Premium	Pieces Iris	TAVConnect	Unite Us
Resource Directory									
Type	Comprehensive	Focused	Focused	Comprehensive	Comprehensive	Comprehensive	Comprehensive	Focused	Focused
Vetting	Vendor, with input on additional resources by customer, CBO, or end users	Customer	Customer	Vendor, with additional inclusion criteria suggested by customer	Vendor and customer	Vendor and customer	Customer and vendor	Customer and vendor	Customer and vendor
Maintenance	By vendor; every 180 days	By participating organizations and by network administrator, as needed	By participating organizations, as needed	By vendor; every 90 - 180 days.	By vendor; every 180 days	By vendor every 180 days for most	By participating organizations as needed and by vendor every 180 days	By vendor every 180 days	Ongoing by participating organizations or coordination center
User flagging	Yes	Yes	No	Yes	Yes	Yes	Yes	Yes	Yes
Screening									
Built-in social needs screening tools	PRAPARE, AHC, and more	No	Yes	PRAPARE, AHC, WE CARE, Healthify proprietary tool, and more	PRAPARE, AHC, and more	4 domain-specific tools	Question bank by domain	Vendor-designed screening tool; PRAPARE; library of 120+ assessments	PRAPARE, AHC, Health Leads, DPP, proprietary tool; others supported
Customization	Yes	Yes	Yes	Yes	Yes	Yes	Yes	Yes	Yes
Responsive recommendations	Yes	No	Yes	Yes	Yes	Yes	Yes	Yes	Yes
Search Options									
Categories	10 major categories 300+ service types Created and uses Open Eligibility taxonomy	Custom categories and service types	Custom categories and service types	13 major categories 326 service types 121 eligibility types Open Referral interoperable	23 major categories 250 service types	9 service areas, categories 200+ granular tags Created and uses Social Services Data Standards	25 customizable categories - also by service types	Uses AIRS taxonomy	20 major categories 150+ service types Mapped to AIRS taxonomy, ICD-10 Z codes, and Open Referral Interoperable.
Search fields	Coverage area, Service Category, Free-text search, including service description, service name, provider name, etc. Additional search tool configuration.	Service category, Service provider name, Service description	Location, Service provider name, Service description	Location, Search radius, Service Category, Eligibility Category, Regional Results, Preferred Status, Network Status	Location, Search radius, Service Category, Condition algorithms	Location, Service provider name, Need, Service description, Service category, Program eligibility, Hours of operation. Additional custom search fields where relevant.	Program name, Need, Service category	Social category, Location, Service area, Eligibility criteria, and others	Service Category, Location, Search Radius, Program Eligibility, Hours of operation. Additional custom search fields where relevant.
Filters	200+ filters	2 filters	10+ filters	6 filters	11 filters	5 filters	3 filters	10 filters	10 filters
User favorites	Yes	No	Yes	Yes	Yes	Yes	Yes	Yes	Yes
End users	Staff Public	Staff Public (add-on fee)	Staff	Staff Patients (through API integration with Patient/Member portal) Public (white-labeled site)	Staff Patients	Public Patients Staff	Staff	Staff Patients (in app, web portal, and/or API integration with patient/member portal)	Staff Patients Public

Figure 11-4. Screenshot Excerpt from *Community Resource Referral Platforms: A Guide for Health Care Organizations* From the Social Interventions Research & Evaluation Network[a]

[a] Platform specifications are changing rapidly over time. Aunt Bertha is now FindHelp. Unite Us purchased NowPow, now combined under Unite Us.

AHC indicates accountable health community; AIRS, Alliance of Information & Referral Systems; API, application programming interface; CBO, community-based organization; DPP, Diabetes Prevention Program; ICD-10, *International Classification of Diseases, 10th Revision;* PRAPARE, Protocol for Responding to and Assessing Patients' Assets, Risks and Experience; and WE CARE, Well Child Care, Evaluation, Community Resources, Advocacy, Referral, Education.

From Cartier Y, Fichtenberg C, Gottlieb L. *Community Resource Referral Platforms: A Guide for Health Care Organizations.* Social Interventions Research & Evaluation Network; 2019. Accessed May 6, 2024. https://sirenetwork.ucsf.edu/tools-resources/resources/community-resource-referral-platforms-guide-health-care-organizations.

Some have also argued that screening for social needs in isolation, without an accompanying ability to provide appropriate resources in response, is ineffective and unethical.[31] Effectively linking patients with community resources to address social needs within many possible domains (eg, food, housing, transportation, education, employment) requires multidisciplinary collaboration with social service professionals and cross-sector collaboration with CBOs that many health care facilities may not yet have established. Screening without adequate response to addressing resulting needs could leave patients frustrated with unfulfilled expectations. Patients could perceive clinicians to be "screening for the sake of screening," or to potentially be using screening results to judge and stigmatize, which could significantly weaken therapeutic relationships.

It is heartening to know, however, that there is another side to all of this. Researchers have demonstrated through qualitative studies that screening for social needs can have benefits apart from any subsequent social care intervention.[32,33] Clinicians can gain a deeper understanding of their patients' social contexts and concerns through screening, allowing for more tailored and comprehensive care. For example, if a patient has difficulty with transportation, their health care team may make a more concerted effort to cluster all medical appointments on one day. If a patient has housing instability, health care professionals may avoid prescribing a medication that requires refrigeration. And so forth. Socially tailored care has the potential to improve the appropriateness and effectiveness of other medical interventions prescribed. In addition, screening for social needs can facilitate more in-depth discussions about patients' social context. Patients have reported that they don't necessarily expect medical teams to be able to resolve their social issues but instead, through conversation, want their clinicians to understand, express empathy, and validate their lived experiences.[32] If patients feel understood and supported by these conversations, screening for social needs could strengthen rather than weaken the patient-clinician relationship. Finally, if social needs screening is made routine and universally performed, patients are less likely to feel targeted, singled out, or judged. By making screening and conversations about social circumstance the norm in health care settings, clinicians may destigmatize the whole screening and referral process for patients, thereby also destigmatizing the use of social services.

Key Concept

Performing screening without an adequate ability to address identified social needs has the potential for both unintended negative consequences (eg, unfulfilled family expectations and erosion of trust in the health care system) and positive consequences (eg, socially tailored care, validation of patients' lived experiences). How screening is ultimately received by families will depend on their personal lived experiences and the empathy and humility with which we approach these sensitive conversations.

Future Directions

Where do we go from here? What approaches might we take to integrate social care into clinical practice in a way that is feasible and effective while avoiding the potential for unintended negative consequences?

In the past, effective social care programs within clinical settings have included standardized social needs screening paired with premade resource handouts tailored to the local community, social work referral to identify relevant resources, and/or referral to an in-person CHW or patient navigator to facilitate referrals and longer-term care.[11,13,17] Although effective, these approaches may not be feasible in health care settings with large catchment populations (ie, it would be impossible to have knowledge of all patients' local community resources) or with limited resource and/or personnel availability to implement screening or address identified needs. If we are to truly make social care an integral part of routine medical care at a large scale and do so in a way that is acceptable and most helpful for families, we must develop innovative ways to overcome barriers and improve screening and referral processes to optimize pediatric health and advance health equity.

Information Technology Innovations

In the early 21st century, advancements made in hardware, software, encryption, artificial intelligence, and the internet are unprecedented. Health care has derived much benefit from this technology revolution, from robotics to predictive modeling and beyond. More broadly, as part of the American Recovery and Reinvestment Act signed in 2009, all public and private health care entities were required to adopt an EHR. Although many clinicians may have data input woes associated with the rise of EHRs, it is undeniable that the universal use of electronic health systems has revolutionized health care's ability to track, report, and share data and to implement electronic interventions. Now and into the distant future, we can capitalize on these technological advancements to improve and expand social care within clinical practice.

Resource Referral Platforms

Through the years, multiple online or app-based social resource referral platforms have been developed, tested, and launched. These platforms (eg, CharityTracker, CrossTx, FindHelp, Healthify, Unite Us) use patients' zip codes to identify local community resources.[28] This approach to resource referral may become particularly useful for either health care systems with larger catchment populations (eg, academic medical centers, children's hospitals), for which it would be difficult to create community resource handouts that were relevant to all patients, or systems with limited or no social service support. Some EHR vendors are now partnering with particular social resource referral platforms, offering integration of the platform into the EHR as part of their most premium packages, and closed-loop referral options to be able to visualize within the EHR when a patient has ultimately received a resource or social service. Although having many desirable properties, these integrated EHR-referral platform models are currently limited and expensive, which may preclude use for many health care systems. But if we develop more EHR-platform partnerships and think innovatively about how to integrate these technology-based platforms into our EHRs and patient gateways while maintaining patient privacy, we may drive down cost and overcome financial barriers to use. Through more use of these integrated models, we could potentially overcome health care systems' own resource/personnel barriers and connect more families to relevant community resources. Additionally, this approach could have positive implications for data tracking for quality metrics, and for research to more easily identify positive health outcomes associated with screening and referral, that could be derived directly from the EHR.

If financial barriers associated with integrated EHR-referral platform models cannot be overcome, some referral platforms also offer free web-based versions that do not allow for any closed-loop referral communication but otherwise contain the same breadth of zip code–based community resource information. Some states have a 211 resource platform available both online and via telephone. Text messaging, QR codes, or web-based links embedded into clinical documentation can also be considered to deliver the referral platform and its wealth of resource information to our patients and families without incurring substantial cost to the health care system.

Tele-Navigation

Although technology-based referral platforms have many benefits and desirable properties, they may also be viewed as less personal, lacking human connection, as their use requires little (or even no) patient-clinician interface. Research has shown that linking families with screening-identified social needs to in-person patient navigators, who facilitate access to social services and resources, can resolve families' social needs and improve parent-reported child health.[13] But many health care systems, along with many pediatric primary care practices, may lack funding, personnel, and/or expertise required for patient navigators.

An outcome of the COVID-19 pandemic has been the rise of telemedicine and payment models that allow telehealth to be a more feasible clinical care delivery option. We can learn from the pandemic to develop innovative and more feasible approaches to social care delivery within clinical care. In the future, health care systems may consider the use of tele-navigators to deliver resource referral interventions to families with identified social needs. Tele-navigators may represent a more fiscally conservative option for health care systems than in-person navigators, and their use could also overcome constraints in personnel availability and/or clinical schedules. The virtual delivery option may allow for more individuals to become patient navigators who may otherwise face barriers to regular travel to a clinic or hospital. By increasing the navigation workforce, tele-navigation may also create more opportunity for families in need to be connected to navigators from their own communities, or with their own racial and ethnic backgrounds, engendering greater trust between the family and navigator as they discuss sensitive social topics. If tele-navigation can build stronger relationships between families and navigators, it has the potential to be even more effective than in-person navigation to resolve social needs and improve child health.

Key Concept

The information technology revolution provides a ripe environment to develop and/or implement innovative technology-supported interventions to help make social care within clinical practice more feasible, sustainable, acceptable, and effective.

Considering Digital Inequity

Information technology innovations will inevitably be a cornerstone of social care growth within clinical medicine. It is vital, however, that we keep health equity at the forefront of our minds as more digital advancements are developed, tested, and implemented. How do we advance health equity in the face of these technological advancements? We must consider our patient populations and their resources. If we assume patients have access to the internet and technology to deliver our social care interventions, we run the risk of worsening disparities through unequal access to or use of these effective interventions. Health care systems may therefore consider use of multi-modality delivery options for social care interventions to ensure equal opportunity for all patients.

Incorporating an Anti-Racist Lens

Structural racism and discrimination are unfortunately part of US history and have become interwoven into our societal structures, which have continually reinforced limitation of opportunities and resources for groups that have been historically marginalized. This has led to disparities in health and adverse SDOH, particularly for people of color.[34,35] Unfortunately, in the United States, such health disparities are only increasing over time. This trend has been particularly salient since 2020, with the majority of children in the United States from racially and ethnically marginalized groups (ie, we have a "minority majority" of children).[36]

In theory, screening for and addressing social needs should reduce child health inequities and disparities by fostering balance in health opportunities and ensuring that more families have consistent access to needs required for basic living. This is one of the motivations for the AAP and the AAFP policy statements recommending screening for and addressing adverse SDOH at all child health encounters. But research has shown that even though social needs screening and referral systems do, in fact, increase social service referrals and family receipt of resources, families of color are more likely to experience a double loss, in which they disclose unmet social needs but do not have their needs addressed.[37,38]

These experiences of double loss may be caused by discrimination and implicit bias at multiple levels of health care and multiple stages of the screening and referral process. Performance of social needs screening, even if meant to be universal and delivered in the exact same way for each patient without judgment, could be influenced by clinicians' implicit biases. If a caregiver has experienced prior trauma from racism or has a negative experience with screening caused by perceived biases, they may be less likely to disclose needs to receive help or may be less likely to engage in downstream referral processes for fear of negative judgment. Prior research has also demonstrated that groups that have been racially and ethnically marginalized experience greater stigma and barriers within the medical and social service systems, which may preclude receipt of resources for caregivers of color.[39,40]

Key Concept

When clinicians are implementing social care screening and referral interventions, people of color are more likely to experience discrimination and implicit biases. This likelihood is caused by structural and multilevel racism in our health care system and social services that must be mitigated through active anti-racism efforts.

As we continue to develop, adapt, and evolve social needs screening and referral processes within clinical care, it is imperative that we incorporate an anti-racist lens at all stages (**Figure 11-5**). We must engage caregivers of color to determine their perceptions on how to best indiscriminately screen, how clinicians should approach discussions about racism and adverse SDOH when needs are disclosed, what barriers they encounter to referrals and accessing resources, and

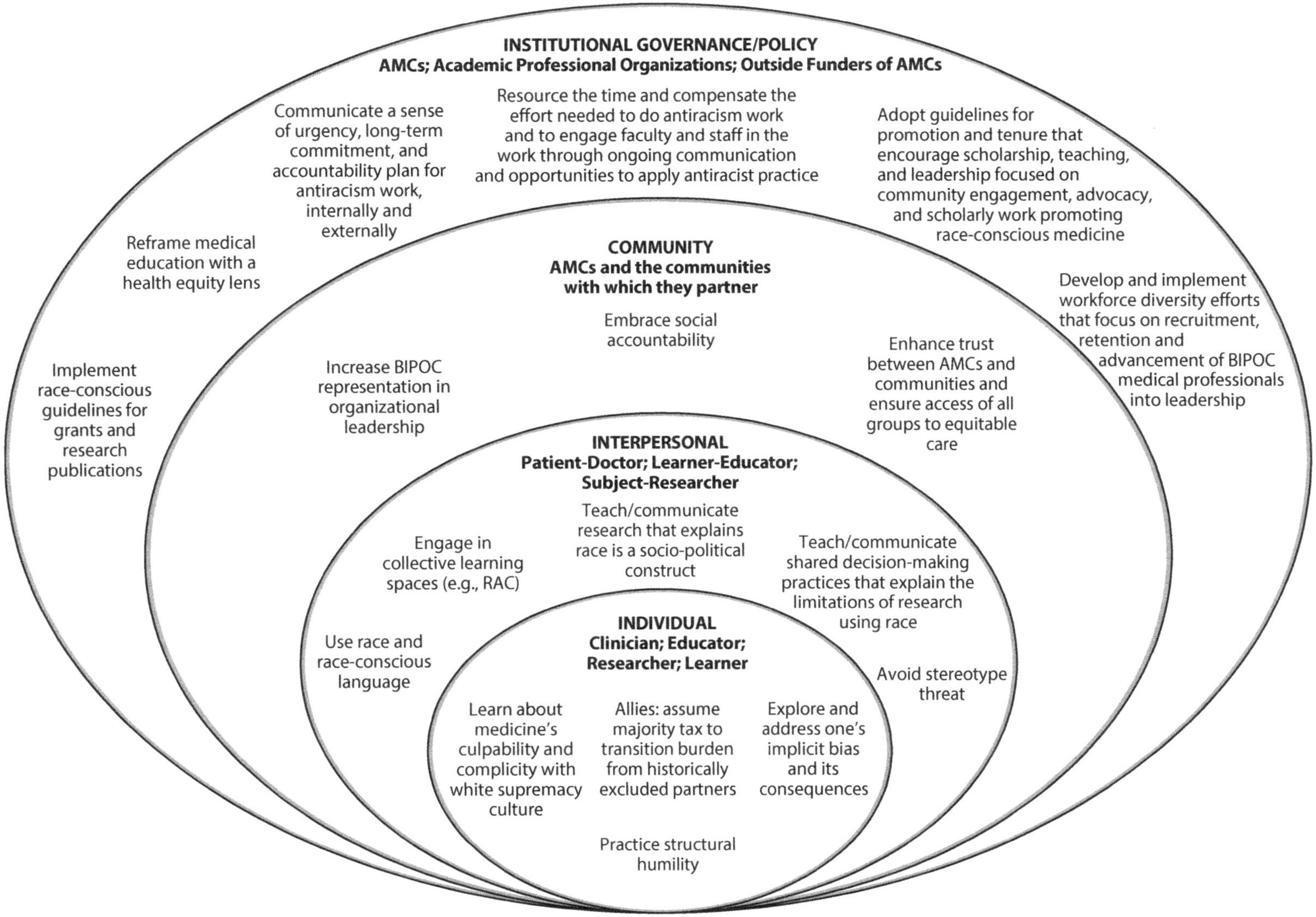

Figure 11-5. A Socioecological Framework for Addressing and Dismantling the Legacy of Race and Racism in Academic Medicine

AMC indicates academic medical center; BIPOC, Black, Indigenous, and people of color; and RAC, racial-affinity caucusing.

From Edgoose JYC, Carvajal DN, Reavis KMP, Yogendran L, Echiverri AT, Rodriguez JE. Addressing and dismantling the legacy of race and racism in academic medicine: a socioecological framework. *J Am Board Fam Med*. 2022;35(6):1239–1245.

what changes they believe could be made to our health care systems, social service agencies, and policies to facilitate their receipt of services and community resources. Such engagement is not easy. It takes a lot of planning and can be time consuming. But it is imperative if we want our social care implementation efforts to be successful for and beneficial to all families, particularly those most marginalized in society. If we incorporate an anti-racist lens into our current and future social needs screening and referral implementation efforts, only then may we be capable of improving child health equity and reducing health and developmental disparities.

Conclusion

The goal of integrating social care into clinical practice goes well beyond simply screening a patient via a piece of paper (or a computer/tablet) and making a referral. It's ultimately about our connections with patients and families. It's about creating a safe environment with meaningful relationships so families feel comfortable sharing their basic needs despite the possible stigma associated, deepening our therapeutic relationships. It is on us as clinicians to show compassion through families' vulnerabilities, to be empathetic and validate their lived experiences, and then to facilitate helpful connections to resources in their communities. We must learn how to embed this process into our daily work in a way that is acceptable to families, feasible, and appropriate within our clinical workflows and time demands, so it can truly be made universal practice. Only then will screening and referring for social needs become part of the fabric and culture of clinical care, performed universally without assumptions or judgment. If this process is also performed with an anti-racist lens, we could ultimately connect historically marginalized populations to community resources more equitably.

In the short-term, we must listen to our families through the conversations following screening, acknowledge their lived experiences in those vulnerable moments, and then do our very best to refer and provide support. But in the longer term, we must advocate for better social policies that will grow and sustain a robust social safety net in the United States and alleviate child poverty. In doing all of this, we can make health care a piece of the solution to reduce disparities and achieve child health equity.

Key Points

Clinicians can make a positive impact on patients' adverse SDOH by

- Advocating for state and federal policy interventions and investments in the broader social safety net, which are known to be effective in lifting children out of poverty and improving child health and development
- Partnering with clinical colleagues and families to develop social needs screening and referral strategies that are tailored to our local clinical environments' resources, making the strategies more acceptable, sustainable, patient centered, and effective
- Creating partnerships with CBOs that have long-standing expertise in local resources and leveraging technology innovations and referral platforms to strengthen and expand the reach of our social care in clinical settings
- Approaching each conversation about social needs screening and individual patient's social needs with empathy and humility, validating our patients' lived experiences, and forging a path together for socially tailored care
- Making active efforts to dismantle racism in all levels of health care and pursue systemic equality

References

1. Child poverty. UNICEF. Accessed May 6, 2024. https://www.unicef.org/social-policy/child-poverty
2. Shrider EA, Creamer J. Poverty in the United States: 2022. US Census Bureau. September 12, 2023. Accessed May 6, 2024. https://www.census.gov/library/publications/2023/demo/p60-280.html
3. American Academy of Pediatrics Council on Community Pediatrics. Poverty and child health in the United States. *Pediatrics.* 2016;137(4):e20160339 PMID: 26962238 doi: 10.1542/peds.2016-0339
4. Hoynes HW, Miller DL, Simon D. The EITC: linking income to real health outcomes. *Center for Poverty Research Policy Brief.* 1(2) doi: 10.15141/S5SG6Q
5. Burns K, Fox L, Wilson D. Expansions to Child Tax Credit contributed to 46% decline in child poverty since 2020. US Census Bureau. September 13, 2022. Accessed May 6, 2024. https://www.census.gov/library/stories/2022/09/record-drop-in-child-poverty.html
6. Duncan GJ, Ziol-Guest KM, Kalil A. Early-childhood poverty and adult attainment, behavior, and health. *Child Dev.* 2010;81(1):306–325 PMID: 20331669 doi: 10.1111/j.1467-8624.2009.01396.x
7. Perry CD, Kenney GM. Preventive care for children in low-income families: how well do Medicaid and state children's health insurance programs do? *Pediatrics.* 2007;120(6):e1393–e1401 PMID: 18055657 doi: 10.1542/peds.2006-3520
8. Jackson MI. Early childhood WIC participation, cognitive development and academic achievement. *Soc Sci Med.* 2015;126:145–153 PMID: 25555255 doi: 10.1016/j.socscimed.2014.12.018
9. Accountable care organizations (ACOs): general information. Centers for Medicare & Medicaid Services. Accessed May 6, 2024. https://innovation.cms.gov/innovation-models/aco
10. Garg A, Butz AM, Dworkin PH, Lewis RA, Thompson RE, Serwint JR. Improving the management of family psychosocial problems at low-income children's well-child care visits: the WE CARE Project. *Pediatrics.* 2007;120(3):547–558 PMID: 17766528 doi: 10.1542/peds.2007-0398
11. Garg A, Toy S, Tripodis Y, Silverstein M, Freeman E. Addressing social determinants of health at well child care visits: a cluster RCT. *Pediatrics.* 2015;135(2):e296–e304 PMID: 25560448 doi: 10.1542/peds.2014-2888
12. Gold R, Bunce A, Cowburn S, et al. Adoption of social determinants of health EHR tools by community health centers. *Ann Fam Med.* 2018;16(5):399–407 PMID: 30201636 doi: 10.1370/afm.2275
13. Gottlieb LM, Hessler D, Long D, et al. Effects of social needs screening and in-person service navigation on child health. *JAMA Pediatr.* 2016;170(11):e162521 PMID: 27599265 doi: 10.1001/jamapediatrics.2016.2521
14. Sokol R, Austin A, Chandler C, et al. Screening children for social determinants of health: a systematic review. *Pediatrics.* 2019;144(4):e20191622 PMID: 31548335 doi: 10.1542/peds.2019-1622
15. Garg A, Brochier A, Tripodis Y, Messmer E, Drainoni ML. A social care system implemented in pediatric primary care: a cluster RCT. *Pediatrics.* 2023;152(2):e2023061513 PMID: 37492934 doi: 10.1542/peds.2023-061513
16. Colvin JD, Bettenhausen JL, Anderson-Carpenter KD, Collie-Akers V, Chung PJ. Caregiver opinion of in-hospital screening for unmet social needs by pediatric residents. *Acad Pediatr.* 2016;16(2):161–167 PMID: 26946270 doi: 10.1016/j.acap.2015.06.002
17. Colvin JD, Bettenhausen JL, Anderson-Carpenter KD, et al. Multiple behavior change intervention to improve detection of unmet social needs and resulting resource referrals. *Acad Pediatr.* 2016;16(2):168–174 PMID: 26183003 doi: 10.1016/j.acap.2015.06.001
18. Lopez MA, Yu X, Hetrick R, et al. Social needs screening in hospitalized pediatric patients: a randomized controlled trial. *Hosp Pediatr.* 2023;13(2):95–114 PMID: 36594231 doi: 10.1542/hpeds.2022-006815

19. Fortin K, Vasan A, Wilson-Hall CL, Brooks E, Rubin D, Scribano PV. Using quality improvement and technology to improve social supports for hospitalized children. *Hosp Pediatr.* 2021;11(10):1120–1129 PMID: 34475224 doi: 10.1542/hpeds.2020-005800

20. Gottlieb LM, DeSilvey SC, Fichtenberg C, Bernheim S, Peltz A. Developing national social care standards. *Health Affairs Forefront* blog. February 22, 2023. Accessed May 6, 2024. https://www.healthaffairs.org/content/forefront/developing-national-social-care-standards

21. Garg A, Homer CJ, Dworkin PH. Addressing social determinants of health: challenges and opportunities in a value-based model. *Pediatrics.* 2019;143(4):e20182355 PMID: 30902829 doi: 10.1542/peds.2018-2355

22. Alley DE, Asomugha CN, Conway PH, Sanghavi DM. Accountable health communities—addressing social needs through Medicare and Medicaid. *N Engl J Med.* 2016;374(1):8–11 PMID: 26731305 doi: 10.1056/NEJMp1512532

23. Bauer MS, Damschroder L, Hagedorn H, Smith J, Kilbourne AM. An introduction to implementation science for the non-specialist. *BMC Psychol.* 2015;3(1):32 PMID: 26376626 doi: 10.1186/s40359-015-0089-9

24. The Health Leads Screening Toolkit. Health Leads. Accessed May 6, 2024. https://healthleadsusa.org/news-resources/the-health-leads-screening-toolkit

25. PRAPARE. National Association of Community Health Centers. March 20, 2023. Accessed May 6, 2024. https://www.nachc.org/prapare

26. Kenyon C, Sandel M, Silverstein M, Shakir A, Zuckerman B. Revisiting the social history for child health. *Pediatrics.* 2007;120(3):e734–e738 PMID: 17766513 doi: 10.1542/peds.2006-2495

27. Billioux A, Verlander K, Anthony S, Alley D. Standardized screening for health-related social needs in clinical settings: the Accountable Health Communities screening tool. *NAM Perspect.* 2017 doi: 10.31478/201705b

28. Cartier Y, Fichtenberg C, Gottlieb L. *Community Resource Referral Platforms: A Guide for Health Care Organizations.* Social Interventions Research & Evaluation Network; 2019. Accessed May 6, 2024. https://sirenetwork.ucsf.edu/tools-resources/resources/community-resource-referral-platforms-guide-health-care-organizations

29. The EveryONE Project Toolkit. American Academy of Family Physicians. Accessed May 6, 2024. https://www.aafp.org/family-physician/patient-care/the-everyone-project/toolkit.html

30. Social Interventions Research & Evaluation Network. Evidence & Resource Library. Accessed May 6, 2024. https://sirenetwork.ucsf.edu/tools/evidence-library

31. Garg A, Boynton-Jarrett R, Dworkin PH. Avoiding the unintended consequences of screening for social determinants of health. *JAMA.* 2016;316(8):813–814 PMID: 27367226 doi: 10.1001/jama.2016.9282

32. Byhoff E, De Marchis EH, Hessler D, et al. Part II: a qualitative study of social risk screening acceptability in patients and caregivers. *Am J Prev Med.* 2019;57(6)(suppl 1):S38–S46 PMID: 31753278 doi: 10.1016/j.amepre.2019.07.016

33. Byhoff E, Gottlieb LM. When there is value in asking: an argument for social risk screening in clinical practice. *Ann Intern Med.* 2022;175(8):1181–1182 PMID: 35696689 doi: 10.7326/M22-0147

34. Marmot M. Social determinants of health inequalities. *Lancet.* 2005;365(9464):1099–1104 PMID: 15781105 doi: 10.1016/S0140-6736(05)71146-6

35. World Health Organization. Social determinants of health. Accessed October 8, 2024. https://www.who.int/health-topics/social-determinants-of-health#tab=tab_1

36. Menchaca A, Pratt B, Jensen E, Jones N; Population Division. Examining the racial and ethnic diversity of adults and children. US Census Bureau. May 22, 2023. Accessed May 6, 2024. https://www.census.gov/newsroom/blogs/random-samplings/2023/05/racial-ethnic-diversity-adults-children.html

37. Schleifer D, Diep A, Grisham K. It's about trust: parents' perspectives on pediatricians screening for social needs. United Hospital Fund. Accessed May 6, 2024. https://uhfnyc.org/publications/publication/its-about-trust-SDH

38. Brochier A, Messmer E, Tripodis Y, Drainoni ML, Garg A. Racial and ethnic inequities in families' receipt of referrals for unmet social needs in pediatric primary care. Poster presented at: Pediatric Academic Societies Meeting; 2022; Denver, CO

39. Young AS, Rabiner D. Racial/ethnic differences in parent-reported barriers to accessing children's health services. *Psychol Serv*. 2015;12(3):267–273 PMID: 25602502 doi: 10.1037/a0038701

40. Hall WJ, Chapman MV, Lee KM, et al. Implicit racial/ethnic bias among health care professionals and its influence on health care outcomes: a systematic review. *Am J Public Health*. 2015;105(12):e60–e76 PMID: 26469668 doi: 10.2105/AJPH.2015.302903

Index

Page numbers followed by *f* indicate figures.